MINDFULNESS IN SCHOOLS
MANUAL

JENNY KIERSTEAD
BLAIR ABBASS

YOGA

BreathingSpace
YOGA STUDIO

Cover Image Michal Bednarek via www.shutterstock.com
Cover Design and Interior Design by Woven Red Author Services, www.WovenRed.ca

Permission granted for the reproduction of the following articles:
Kelly Mahler, Interoception; "The Eighth Sense"
Leah Kuypers, "The Zones of Regulation"
David A. Treleaven, "Trauma-Sensitive Mindfulness"
Micheal Meade, "The Story of the Firebird"

Mindfulness in Schools Manual/Jenny Kierstead, Blair Abbass—1st edition
ISBN student manual paperback: 978-0-9953409-5-4

Contact Jenny and Blair at:
info@BreathingSpaceYogaStudio.ca
www.YogaInSchools.ca
1 (902)-444-9642

CONTENTS

INTRODUCTION

THE EAGLE

There is old fable about a farmer who discovered an eagle's egg in his field one day. He placed the egg in his chicken coup where it eventually hatched with a brood of chicks. The only reality the eagle had was his community of chickens, so he grew up clucking and cackling and digging in the soil for worms and insects like all the other chickens.

One day, the eagle noticed several large and glorious birds soaring overhead. He asked one of his chicken friends, "Who are they?"

The chicken replied, "Those are eagles, the most magnificent of all birds." The land-bound eagle said dreamily, "Wouldn't it be wonderful to fly like that?" The chicken quickly replied, "It's pointless to dream like that, you and I are farm chickens, and this is where we belong."

So, the eagle put his dream of soaring high in the sky out of his head and lived out his days as a well-behaved barnyard chicken.

Life today is very different from what it was even fifty years ago. With constant access to our mobile devices and an infinite library at our fingertips, we are provided with information that could easily fill our minds 24 hours a day, each day of our lives. We're not that far off, with the latest research showing that teens are on the screen an average of seven to nine hours a day—that's more time than they spend at school!

Advances in technology have indeed revealed solutions to many former life-threatening diseases and struggles. These advances, however, have occurred at such rapid speed that their power has almost exceeded our ability to skillfully incorporate them into our lives in a safe, healthy and balanced way.

In terms of our potential as human beings, many of us are so deeply entranced in the many distractions available today or confined by a crippling perspective of ourselves that we're stuck in the chicken coup, like the eagle in the story above, without ever realizing just how much awesomeness we actually possess.

Moreover, in efforts to be productive and lucrative in our lives while providing our children with as many life experiences as possible, we've created a culture of chaotic movement and obsessive busy-ness. After some distressing research results, we are now pausing to ask ourselves if we are indeed evolving or recklessly stumbling into our future with our heads in our phones.

Given the stress related disorders that plague our populations, from the young to the elderly, it is clear to see that we need help in striking a new balance, one that harmoniously incorporates all the components of our new world lifestyle. Enter the practice of mindfulness, which is proving to be a significant benefactor in our attempt to achieve a new set point of health and well-being amidst the new demands on our time.

Why is mindfulness catching so many people's attention? Because it's simple, effective and applicable to everyone. Regardless of your age, race or status, mindfulness works.

Simply put, mindfulness is the process by which we develop the capacity to control our attention. Wouldn't you love to have the ability to focus your full attention on what you want and then shift your attention to another topic when you're ready?

> Attention is like a spotlight and what it illuminates, streams into your mind and shapes your brain. Developing greater control over your attention is perhaps the single most powerful way to reshape your brain and thus your mind.
>
> Rick Hanson, *Buddha's Brain*

Welcome Message from the Authors

I, Blair Abbass, have taught mindfulness within the classroom throughout my thirty-five-year teaching career and I've witnessed stress levels and related health conditions of students and teachers rise to unmanageable heights. While the sources of stress may have changed over the years, stress is still threatening our physical and mental health and young people seem to be especially eager to learn about these contemplative practices.

The mindfulness tools I offered twenty-five years ago to help students deal with exam stress boast the same benefits for students today dealing with technology overload. After years of leading professional development workshops to teachers, I am thrilled to finally have these time-tested methods of stress reduction and life skills compiled in one place.

I, Jenny Kierstead, began my inward journey in my teens in a desperate attempt to heal my mind-body disconnect following a series of traumas. After many painful years of struggle with an eating disorder, my quest for mental health, physical wellbeing and spiritual awakening have remained a fascination at the forefront of my life Now an educator and author with over 10,000 hours of study in yoga and mindfulness from many great wisdom teachers such as Deepak Chopra, Jack Kornfield and Rick Hanson, I feel immensely honored to be a part of this essential field of work.

Throughout our 15 years of bringing our Yoga in Schools programs to teachers and students, we have met a number of trail-blazing leaders who are enhancing the lives of children with their ground breaking, culturally diverse work. It is our privilege to have contributions from the following people included in our manual.

- Kelly Mahler, Interoception Specialist and author of "Interoception; The Eighth Sense"
- Leah Kuypers, author of "The Zones of Regulation"
- David A. Treleaven, author of "Trauma-Sensitive Mindfulness"
- Kelly Humphreys, School Psychologist and Mindfulness Teacher
- Dr. Maria Patriquin, Family Physician and Mindfulness Specialist
- Catherine Rahey, Autism Consultant and Mindfulness Specialist for Autism
- Janean Marshall and Beverely Jeddore, First Nations Leaders in Mi'kmaw Language, Education and Mindfulness Services, MK Board
- Talia Carin, Art therapist (AT), Canadian Certified Counsellor (CCC), Naturotherapist (ND) and Registered Yoga Teacher
- Krishinda McBride, Mindfulness and Drumming Teacher, Coordinator of Race Relations Cross Cultural Understanding and human Rights AVRCE

May this manual help to relieve our children's suffering and propel all of us into greater states of awareness, peace and happiness.

Jenny Kierstead and *Blair Abbass*

We're all seeking the rapture of being alive.
That's what it's all finally about.

Joseph Campbell

The Four Pillars of the Mindfulness Manual

The Mindfulness in Schools Manual is divided into four pillars
1) The practice of mindfulness
2) Movement/somatic practices.
3) Cognitive therapy
4) Story telling

The mindfulness section includes a six-week program, which could be followed if there is an allotted time booked for such a program. The remaining content can be used as reference material and activities within other classes, as a way of infusing mindfulness into students' lives throughout their day. There are various teachings, from the science of mindfulness, quick mindful practices for de-stressing, guided visualizations, personal reflection exercises and group activities.

These lessons can be used individually, as appropriate for a particular class needs or they can be used in sequence, starting at the beginning of the mindfulness segment, progressing through to story-telling.

PILLAR 1: THE PRACTICE OF MINDFULNESS

"NOW's all there is, so peaceful and still.
In NOW you don't worry 'bout what's happened or what will.
Cause NOW never ends and NOW's never been,
And all of your answers are waiting for you here, NOW."

Dave Carroll, singer/songwriter

Studies show that 47% of the time, we're not present to life—that's almost half of our life that we're not really living!

Harvard researcher Matt Killingsworth created an app in attempts to answer the question "what makes us happy?" once and for all, and the results have been an eye-opener. According to Mr. Killingworth's data, we're happiest when we are mindful of the moment, and we're least happy when the mind is wandering.

According to Killingsworth, the average person's mind is wandering around 47% of our day—and when the mind wanders we don't feel happy. Spending so much time with the mind wandering makes us vulnerable to depression, stress, anxiety and other negative emotions.

This research isn't new Mindfulness can be traced back thousands of years to ancient practices and traditions More recently, it was introduced in secular applications beginning over 30 years ago through the work of Jon Kabat-Zinn and Mindfulness-Based Stress Reduction (MBSR).

Mindfulness is now used in medicine, psychology, and corporate settings to address illness, pain and stress, among other things. With 40 years of research, 18, 000 studies and more than 40 studies a month coming out on mindfulness, people are really starting to understand its layered benefits and how it really works.

The growing body of research on mindfulness in school-based contexts reveals the following list of core benefits of mindfulness

- Improved concentration and focus
- Greater emotional regulation and sense of calm
- Decreased stress, anxiety and depression
- Enhanced impulse control and self-awareness
- Increased resilience
- Improved ability to respond skillfully to challenges
- Increased empathy, compassion and understanding of others

With evidence such as this, the workforce is slowly becoming more mindful as well. In a new study of more than 85,000 adults, yoga practice among U.S. workers nearly doubled from 2002 to 2012, from 6 percent to 11 percent. Mindfulness rates also increased, from 8 percent to 9.9 percent. [1]

PILLAR 2: HOW MOVEMENT PRACTICES COMPLEMENT MINDFULNESS

With the fullness of our lives, many people unconsciously go through their days without regard for their body, forgetting how important it is to nourish it adequately with food, water, movement, sleep and appreciation. Our body is the vehicle by which we experience the world. Therefore, neglecting our body

- Hinders our health and therefore, also affects our ability to share our gifts
- Restricts our ability to connect with others
- Leads to chronic illness
- Unnecessarily abbreviates our time here on earth

Through the practice of mindfulness, we begin to awaken the wisdom of the body by opening our inner ear to listen to its needs and messages. The movement practices included here are designed to gently reconnect students to the feeling tone within the body through

[1] Kachan D, Olano H, Tannenbaum SL, Annane DW, Mehta A, Arheart KL, et al. Prevalence of Mindfulness Practices in the US Workforce: National Health Interview Survey. Prev Chronic Dis 2017;14:160034. DOI: http://dx.doi.org/10.5888/pcd14.160034

postures that stretch, strengthen and regulate the breath. Moving mindfully helps us all to live life in a more attentive, harmonious and sensitive fashion. In order to attain true mindfulness, there must be harmony between the psyche (mind) and soma (body) which is why movement practices have been included here.

MINDFUL MOVEMENT

Mindful movement is something everybody can do, requiring no equipment or special skills. Even a short movement practice can contribute to our wellbeing by
- Strengthening muscle
- Improving posture
- Increasing flexibility
- Managing weight
- Balancing hormones
- Flushing stress chemicals
- Calming the mind
- Improving our self-esteem
- Fostering mind/body connection

HOW TO APPROACH THE MOVEMENT PRACTICES

Many people today do yoga as a form of exercise to tighten and tone and sweat away pounds. While it may do all of those things, the practice is designed to both push your physical edge with an element of challenge AND create a sense of relaxed, focused awareness.

In the western world, we have stuffed the wisdom tradition of yoga into the same box as our beauty obsessed paradigm and in many instances, yoga is associated with other 'body sculpting' exercises. The true practice of yoga and other ancient energy management techniques are designed to expand our consciousness and assist us in living a fulfilling and peace-centric life.

The goal of our movement practice within the Mindfulness Manual is to anchor our awareness in our body and our breath, moment by moment. As we do that, we familiarize ourselves with sensations and the messages within them. The more we listen, the more we heal, and whenever there's healing, freedom and happiness follow.

If you have thought that you are not fit, firm or toned enough to try yoga, you have been misinformed of the true purpose and intent of the practice. You need not change a thing about yourself before you embark on the journey. Instead, the best way to prepare starts by accepting the invitation to show up on your mat with full acceptance of who you are now, and a commitment to deepening your understanding and compassion for yourself, for others and for life.

In each movement class, your challenge will be to find that sweet spot that balances effort and ease, which we'll call your growing edge. If you practice beneath your edge by not giving enough physically, or by drifting your attention away from the experience, no change will result. If you overdo it and work too hard, you'll exhaust yourself and risk injury.

When you practice breathing and moving within the boundaries of your growing edge, you'll feel nurtured, inspired and energized You know you're on track when you naturally look and feel more alive, healthy, centered and peaceful, and people start asking what you're doing differently.

WHAT CAN I EXPECT?

Each class will begin with a mindfulness practice with breath awareness in an easy sitting pose or lying down pose. Following this opening segment will be warming postures that increase circulation and prepare your body for more challenging (optional) poses that flush toxins and ignite your healing flame. The class will culminate with a cooling or relaxation phase, designed to help you integrate your experience and insights before heading back into your life.

PILLAR 3: HOW COGNITIVE THERAPY COMPLEMENTS MINDFULNESS

Cognitive Therapy is a perfect complement to mindful practices, helping you become more rational and reasonable by balancing emotional reactivity with logic and common sense This segment includes techniques for dealing with emotional dysregulation by helping you gain a greater understanding of emotional triggers, thereby more effectively dealing with stress. The cognitive-based therapy (also known as CBT) section of the manual, you will learn to skillfully guide their minds into a more positive perspective.

By increasing a positive perspective, you will learn to disempower Automatic Negative Thoughts (ANTs) and expect better outcomes in life.

PILLAR 4: THE BENEFITS OF STORY TELLING

Since the beginning of time people have used stories as a means for teaching and passing on wisdom. People have an inherent love for being read or told stories as they awaken our imagination and generate feelings of magic and wonder.

Instead of demanding the intellectual mind to memorize information, story-telling taps into the emotional aspect of the brain, leaving deep memories of the feelings experienced through the stories It improves listening and communication skills, while sharpening social and emotional intelligences.

Story telling is one of the best ways to deliver any lesson, since the concept is linked to an emotion. This enables us to relate to others through our shared emotional experience, which naturally cultivates compassion and empathy.

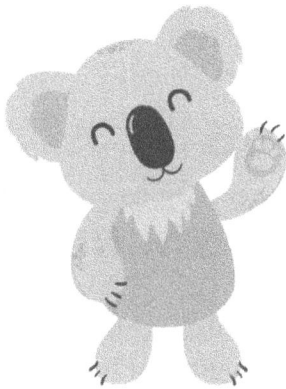

Hello there, my name is Quiet Koala and I'm the Mindfulness in Schools mascot. In our noisy world, I like to fill spaces with a little bit of quiet. Whenever you see me, I'm your reminder to take three deep, relaxing breaths and enjoy a few calm and quiet moments.

Pillar I
Mindfulness

Paying Attention with a Beginner's Mind

A child once thought the word mindfulness referred to a full mind, and he wasn't wrong, since mindfulness helps us to fill our minds with the present moment. But it also helps us to empty our minds, by teaching us to filter out the massive amounts of information we're inundated with on a daily basis. The main goal of mindfulness, however, is neither an empty mind or a full mind, but rather to assume a beginner's mind. When we approach each moment of our lives with a beginner's mind, we view the world with a fresh and new perspective which enables us to learn something from every experience and every encounter.

Mindfulness can be described as the practice of sustaining present moment awareness, on purpose, for a period of time. This doesn't mean that we strive to still our mind, or even empty it, but rather that we return to the present moment over and over again. Through practice, we can even develop the ability to become aware of being aware (also known as meta-cognition). With greater awareness of the moment, we enhance our experience of both our inner world (like our breath, thoughts, emotions, sensations etc) and our outer world (like our seat, the room, our classmates, our city, the earth etc). The neat thing about mindfulness is that this heightened sense of awareness doesn't stop when we close our practice but continues into our daily activities.

Student Reflection

How do you think improving mindful awareness could benefit your life? And the lives of others around you?

Body Benefits

Mindful practices have shown to lessen our experience of chronic stress, which leads to a decrease in cortisol (a major stress hormone responsible for many chronic illnesses such as asthma, heart disease, diabetes, PMS and chronic pain) Lessening stress in our lives naturally boosts our immunity and strengthens our defenses from illness As we decrease our stress and become more aware of our needs, we become better able to care for ourselves. Instead of suddenly being surprised by a health crisis or waiting until an illness is in full expression, we notice an imbalance in its early stages and can deal with it effectively.

STUDENT REFLECTION

After eating your next meal, take notice of how you feel. Does your body feel energized and properly fueled or does your food make you feel sick and drained? Note: if you feel sick or sluggish after eating, consider seeking professional help to individualize your diet.

> Mindfulness has been proven to be one of the few practices that effectively treats ill-health without drug therapy or surgery.
>
> Duncan Armstrong, MD

MIND BENEFITS

Mindfulness has the amazing ability to alter our minds and change our brains. Have you ever considered that your mind and your brain are two different entities? It's true, your mind and brain are not the same. Your mind consists of the invisible activity that includes thoughts, feelings, beliefs, attitudes, knowledge and your imagination. Your brain is the actual organ of the body that resides within your skull, looking similar to a walnut within its shell.

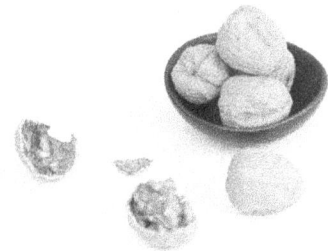

Your brain is associated with your mind and consciousness, but your mind is not restricted to the confines of your brain. In fact, the activity of your mind can affect the cells of your body, not just your brain cells. To prove that your mind has tremendous power over all bodily systems, take a moment to think about something scary, like a tsunami hitting the shores and sweeping everything in its path into the vast ocean. Did you feel that thought in your body? If yes, you might have felt your palms sweat, your throat tighten and your heart start to race. If this continued for a period of time, you might end up holding your breath, becoming constipated and unable to eat. This is known as the stress response, which can be stimulated from a simple thought!

On the contrary, take a moment to think about one of your favourite activities, like bike riding through a nature trail with warm sunlight on your back and green grass brushing your tires. Can you feel that image in your body? If yes, you likely felt a feeling of pleasure flood your system, which caused your jaw and neck to soften, your mouth begin to smile, your breath to deepen, your belly to relax, and your senses begin to tingle. This is the relaxation response, known as rest and digest, which can be awakened by a simple thought!

OUR CHANGING BRAINS

One thing we know about imbalances or habits of any kind, is that the longer they linger, the harder they are to change. That is why mindfulness is so valuable. If your life is a book, your teen years are the first few chapters, making this moment the perfect time for you to be reflecting on your lifestyle habits and how they contribute to your vision for good health, if at all. According to brain researcher Daniel Siegal, the human brain is not fully developed until the mid-twenties, so treating your growing brain with care makes a whole lot of sense.

Consider that the daily practices and habits you engage now may very well set the tone for the rest of your life because the mind and body are drawn to sameness and routine. In fact, most adults are employing the same habits and the same beliefs they've had about themselves since they were children, because they don't realize this most amazing fact: our brains are moldable, like warm clay on a potter's wheel.

Through amazing, cutting-edge brain research, we now know that our brains do not remain the same throughout our lives. Our brains actually change, according to how we nourish them (with food, rest, entertainment, music, practices such as mindful practices and intellectual stimulation) and the life experiences we have. For example, the brain has one hundred billion brain cells, called neurons, and when we undergo an experience, our neurons become active. When neurons fire together, they grow new connections between them. Over time, the connections that result from firing, lead to rewiring in the brain. This is incredibly exciting news because it means that we aren't held captive for the rest of our lives by the way our brain works in this moment—we can actually rewire it so that we can be healthier and happier.[2]

Although the mind and brain are different entities, they influence one another in important ways Our thoughts, known as mental activity, actually shape the pathways of the brain. Repeated mental activity (like a stream of thoughts), leads to repeated brain (neural) activity All of this means that the thoughts we think, over and over, actually shape the form and function of our brains!

The Hebbian Law, taken from Donald Hebb's book 'The organization of behavior' is commonly used to describe this process: neurons that fire together, wire together. In other words, your brain organizes itself according to the focus of your mind. This explains how difficult it is to change an addictive behavior, especially a well-practiced one. But this understanding also explains why repeated practices such as mindfulness can lead to lasting positive changes in our mental health.

STUDENT REFLECTION

Take a few quiet moments to simply watch your thoughts and follow where your mind wanders. What does your mind tend to focus on when it's idling in quiet time? Does the nature of your thoughts contribute to your wellbeing? If not, you now have the power to redirect them with your new-found awareness!

---

[2] Daniel J Seigel MD and Tina Payne Bryson PhD, *The Whole Brain Child* (Bantam Books Trade Paperbacks 2012), 7.

ANATOMY OF THE HUMAN BRAIN

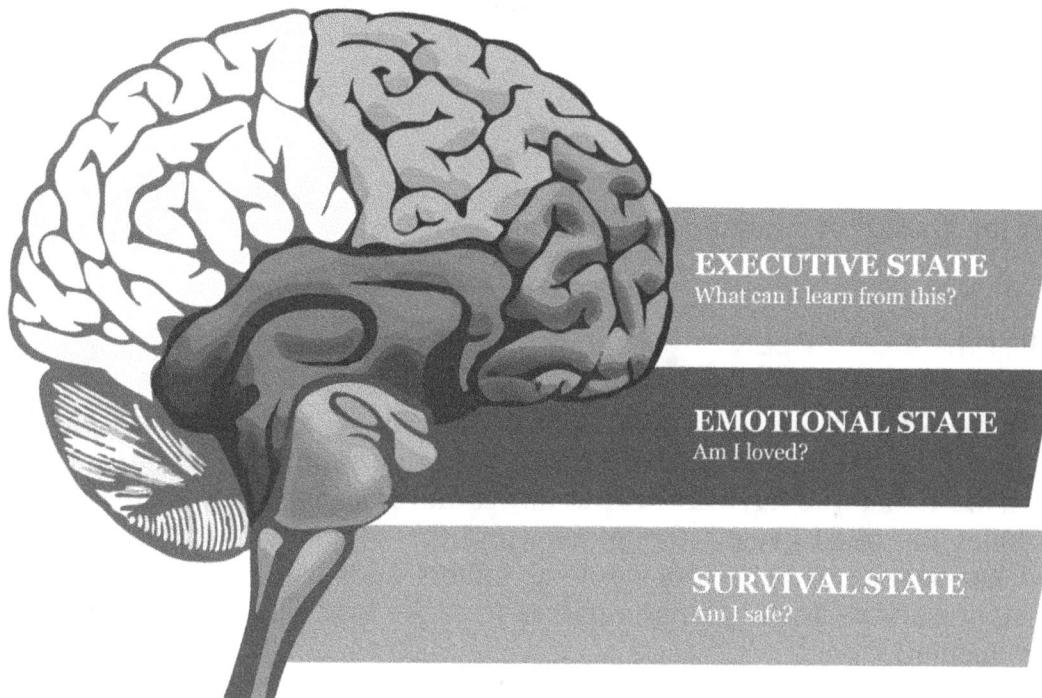

EXECUTIVE STATE
What can I learn from this?

EMOTIONAL STATE
Am I loved?

SURVIVAL STATE
Am I safe?

Let's begin our brief exploration of the brain with a few important facts on neurophysiology, the study of the functioning of the nervous system.

The Autonomic Nervous System (ANS) regulates involuntary bodily functions such as our heart rate and our breathing (which can also be voluntary, as shown in our breathing practices). The ANS also distinguishes between danger and safety with its two branches that work together to either spend or save energy

1. Sympathetic Nervous System, (the gas pedal), activates fight, flight, freeze or flock.
2. Parasympathetic Nervous System, (the brake pedal), allows us to rest, relax and digest.

Our Sympathetic Nervous System (SNS) kicks in when we interpret potential threat or danger, activating our survival-based instincts. In an emergency situation, a blast of energy and stress hormones (adrenalin and cortisol) flood our system, causing blood to surge to our muscles (and away from non-essential functions like digestion) which enables us to fight or flee. A sympathetic reaction gives us super human powers that were previously not available to us, like the examples we hear of parents lifting cars off of children.

This natural instinct to run or fight is critical for flushing stress hormones and dispersing this powerful surge of energy, but in today's world we too often experience an onslaught of stressors without an outlet for the sudden burst of energy, contributing to physical and mental dysregulation. Have you ever panicked or become stressed about a test in the classroom, or a big game that you spent on the bench, and felt the drive to release pent up energy? Our society makes it tough for us to naturally move our bodies when a stressor strikes, because it's considered not socially appropriate. Instead we 'sit still and behave' and bottle it up inside.

Our most primitive survival reaction to a crisis, however, is to 'freeze', also known as dissociation, in which we literally 'play dead' with the hope of tricking our predator into thinking we're already dead. If it doesn't deter the predator, freezing at the very least releases endorphins, numbing us so we can endure the event and hopefully survive.

The brain has three parts, which the late Paul D. MacLean named the truine brain

- The neocortex
- The limbic system
- The reptilian complex

Within these three general parts, there are important components of the brain that are affected by the practice of mindfulness, which are noted below.

THE REPTILIAN COMPLEX

We could think of our brains like a house whose frame is built a certain size and then over the years, receives a few additions. Like a house, the brain is built from the ground up, with the reptilian brain that we share with lizards, turtles and crocs at base of the skull. This region, which includes the basal ganglia, brain stem and the cerebellum, is responsible for the instinctual, survival-based behaviors we do as infants, such as eating, sleeping, breathing, crying, urinating and defecating (often referred to as the four Fs: Feeding, Fighting, Fleeing and...reproduction).

THE RETICULAR ACTIVATING SYSTEM (RAS)

It is almost impossible for our brain to process the millions of sensory stimuli that bombard us at each moment. The Reticular Activating System (RAS), located in the brainstem, does its best to filter this information. This system screens sensory data, allowing only relevant information to pass into our conscious mind.

When we practice mindful awareness, we can more skillfully maintain our focus, and redirect our attention away from unnecessary sensory stimuli toward an intended focal point. This enhances our effectiveness in any project.

Today there are unprecedented demands on our time and attention. We live in an attention economy, with millions of companies, products and websites constantly vying for our attention. Through mindful awareness, we are more consciously able to choose what we want to dedicate our attention to and with that clarity, we can more easily refuse the rest.

THE LIMBIC SYSTEM

A second-floor addition was built right above the reptilian brain, called the mammalian brain, which is similar to other animals who live communally and care for their young. With the hippocampus, amygdala and hypothalamus, it is here that our protective responses like fight/flight/freeze remain on the look-out for both danger and opportunity. Here, our emotional brain has the first say in interpreting incoming stimuli.

Due to this instinct to categorize things, the limbic system is the seat of value-based judgments, which are largely unconscious (until, that is, we take up a mindfulness practice and observe our judging nature).

Within the limbic system is the amygdala, an almond shaped cluster of neurons located deep within the temporal lobes. Known as the 'alarm bell', the amygdala assesses stimuli for danger, with lightning fast reaction time (like within about 1/10th of a second). It reacts to a threat in the following ways

- Fight—like confronting a predator
- Flight—like fleeing from a natural disaster
- Freeze—like holding our breath in shock
- Flock—like running to our caregiver for safety
- Submit—like submitting to an authority figure

For example, seeing a mouse scamper across the floor may signal the amygdala and release adrenalin that then activates an instantaneous whole-body fight/flight reaction. Before you know it, you're on the countertop, climbing toward the window. Which reaction is this an example of? Flight of course.

The human species has survived because of the amygdala's rapid reactivity so it deserves a lot of credit. As a result of its speed, however, it bypasses thinking and goes straight to reacting. The amygdala receives information from our senses and processes social signals, which triggers emotions and leads to action, such as climbing counters in the presence of a rodent.

In a positive situation, information will be sent to the prefrontal cortex for consideration and reasoning. If the information is negative, the SNS kicks in and the amygdala signals arousal centers in the brain to release noradrenalin and adrenalin. These hormones prepare the brain and body to manage a threat and prevent (or slow) information from reaching the prefrontal cortex. It's interesting to note that the amygdala does not distinguish between real or imaginary threats.

Mindfulness has proven to be a successful intervention for calming the amygdala's impulsive reaction to stressful or negative thoughts and experiences so that we can access the pre-frontal cortex (rational, thinking mind) more readily.

The Hippocampus, which means "Sea Horse" in Greek is also part of the limbic system. It is responsible for

- memory (the intentional recall of information)
- registering the nature of situations
- recording the timing of events, giving them a beginning, middle and end.

Our long-term memory has two divisions: implicit and explicit memory. Implicit memory occurs without conscious thought, allowing us to do things automatically, like drive a car or read a book without having to intently focus. Explicit memory requires conscious thought to recall a past experience. The hippocampus records details from past events like the faces of people we know and information learned in school.

But remembering explicit information requires consistent focused attention and when a person is exposed to excessive stress, focus scatters and information is not coded properly. The Hippocampus, which recalls events and lets us know when they've ended, becomes compromised when a stressful state persists. This can not only taint our memories of events but also hinder the message that we can calm down and resume our lives.

The good news is that mindfulness sharpens our attention to the most important information and creates more accurate impressions in our explicit memory, hence improving the learning process.

The insula receives and appraises information about bodily states. It is involved in our ability to sense how we are feeling and to evaluate our emotional well-being. Therefore, the Insula is directly associated with interoception (the ability to inwardly perceive our body's messages. See section on Interoception later in this manual for more information). We know that mindfulness holds the potential to change the structure of the brain, specifically increasing the health and longevity of the Insula, where we engage self-awareness and empathy. When we partake in practices that are designed to cultivate compassion, we actually strengthen the empathetic regions of the brain. Mindfulness has been shown to boost empathy as well as altruistic behaviour.

THE NEOCORTEX

The latest renovation on the house, is the most advanced part of our brain, the neo-cortex, also known as the rational brain. This region allows us to use language, abstract thought, imagination and empathize with others. By age two, our two large hemispheres are developed, and we learn that it's not always in our best interest to react emotionally to every stimuli. Our perspective of life expands and we learn to modify our behaviour in favour of our desires.

The prefrontal cortex (PFC) is the part of the brain that separates us from the rest of the animal kingdom because it enables us to reason, to set goals, to make decisions, to problem solve, to focus and shift our attention and to actually think about thinking (known as self-reflection). The PFC plays a part in shaping our emotions with its ability to direct and restrain the limbic system.

More specifically, the pre-frontal cortex (PFC) which is located just behind the eyes, helps us to rationally assess situations and chart the best course of action. The PFC also helps us to calm down by keeping the emotional brain in check. For example, after realizing you're scaling the walls over a little mouse, you're then able to reason with yourself and climb back down. Receiving information from the hippocampus that an event has passed, the prefrontal cortex enables us to regulate our emotions and restore balance. When we might otherwise react to a trigger, mindfulness instils the practiced ability to stop, breathe (putting the breaks on the amygdala) and think (tapping into the PFC). This goes in opposition to how we are taught to behave in our fast-paced culture that encourages us to go, go, go. Through mindfulness we realize that busy is not always good, or productive, but often a symptom and the cause of chronic stress.

Since mindfulness develops the **prefrontal cortex**, especially the left side where mood enhancement occurs, it makes sense that this practice also leads to more happiness too.

> Studies have shown that as the amygdala shrinks with mindfulness practice, the prefrontal cortex – associated with higher order brain functions such as awareness, concentration and decision-making – becomes thicker.

In other words, with regular mindfulness practice our more primal reactions to stress seem to be replaced by more thoughtful ones.[3]

FROM REACTIVITY TO RESPONSE-ABILITY

Humans are designed as multi-sensory creatures, receiving information from the world around us through our senses of sight, smell, hearing, touch, and taste. This information travels through many levels of processing to eventually create an image in our brain. The way we react to or internalize this image depends on our past life experiences, and our practiced emotional reactions. A typical reaction to a situation would involve a stimulus of some kind (a text message, for example) followed by an instant reaction. Our fast-paced culture today has many people's sympathetic nervous systems running on over-drive, which causes them to jump to conclusions, make rash decisions and react in a state of fight or flight.

STIMULI ~ REACTION

The time between sensory input and our response is delayed when we are mindful of our surroundings and ourselves. Through mindfulness practice, we can learn to observe incoming sensory information before reacting emotionally. If the amygdala responds quickly to a perceived threat, a mindful observer can note the resulting physiological reaction (increased heart and breathing rates), pause and take some breathing space before taking action. This pause allows the prefrontal cortex to reason, prioritize the information, observe one's thoughts and feelings with mindful awareness and then make an appropriate decision.

Taking this time to process the incoming information and consider the consequences leads to more thoughtful action. This powerful understanding enables us to shift from an irrational reaction to a conscious response, leading to behavior choices that are more aligned with the highest vision we hold for ourselves. Over time, with constant practice, this not only leads to better life choices but also a greater ability to regulate emotions. Isn't that exciting?

STIMULI ~ BREATHING SPACE ~ RESPONSE

RBC—an easy acronym to help with this process of creating more breathing space between a situation and your response-ability is to

Relax – relax your mind and body
Breathe – breathe deeply three times (for more details, see the section on breath-regulating practices)

---

[3] Scientific American – "What does mindfulness meditation do to your brain".
https://blogs.scientificamerican.com/guest-blog/what-does-mindfulness-meditation-do-to-your-brain

Choose – when you're able to calm down enough to access your reasoning powers, you can then choose your best course of action

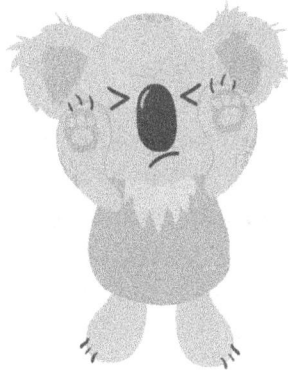

Even bears' brains can experience stress--Relax, Breathe and Choose. Relax, Breathe and Choose.

THE BRAIN'S RESPONSE TO TRAUMA

Extreme emotional states, such as rage, panic or intense fear that arise from traumatic experiences, reduces prefrontal cortex activity, which hampers our ability to think rationally and regulate our behavior. What's more, when the alarm bells continue to sound, stress hormones interfere with the Hippocampus, and the rational brain never gets the message that the event has ended. If the hippocampus remains highjacked and the amygdala stays on overdrive in panic mode, PTSD can develop.

"When the alarm bell of the emotional brain keeps signaling that you are in danger, no amount of insight will silence it" says Bessel van der Kolk. Realizing that some behavioural issues may very well be a sympathetic reaction, stemming from the constant firing of the internal alarm bells within the limbic system is essential awareness to have when implementing mindfulness into our classrooms. It is clear, then, how much caution we must exercise when asking our students to be mindful of sensations in their bodies and streams of thoughts in their minds.

STUDENT REFLECTION

Think of a nonthreatening situation in your own life (like a rodent in the kitchen) when you were startled suddenly, and you reacted impulsively (and unnecessarily) by fleeing, fighting or freezing. Can you see the benefits of learning to calm that reactive nature, allowing you to pause and take a few mindful breaths before taking action?

STUDENT ACTIVITY

1. Research the findings on mindfulness and neuroscience. How does this practice alter and enhance the structures of the brain?

2. Do a search on mindfulness and record five different experts' descriptions of the practice and its benefits. Create a collage on Bristol board with these answers and your own reflections and present it to a small group.

Samples

Mindfulness is paying attention on purpose non-judgmentally in the present moment as if your life depended on it.

Jon Kabat Zinn

Meditation (mindfulness) is the best way to handle stress in your life. This simple practice not only decreases the negative effects of stress, it can actually reverse them.

Deepak Chopra

The ability to voluntarily bring back a wandering attention over and over again is the very root of judgment, character, and will. An education that sharpens one's attention would be education par excellence.

William James, *The Principles of Psychology*

BRAIN WAVE STATES

The human brain is an amazing little organ, averaging about the size of our fist, weighing in at a mere three pounds. Encased in the skull bones, surrounded by cerebrospinal fluid, the brain rests on top of the spinal column to make up our central nervous system. The nervous system controls most of the activity of the body and processes the constant stream of information we receive from our senses. Despite its small size, however, this pint-sized organ is vastly complex with abilities we are still uncovering. One of those discoveries is the knowledge that the brain has various wave speeds or frequencies, which affect our state of being.

STUDENT ACTIVITY

1. Research the different brain sizes of various animals and the capacities that each one possesses. Does brain size indicate intelligence?
2. Do other animals possess the same ability that humans have to self-reflect and observe our own behaviour?
3. Do other species have various brain wave frequencies too?

Did you know that your brain has five different speeds? They are called: **Beta, alpha, theta, delta and gamma.** Each frequency is measured in cycles per second (Hz) and has its own set of characteristics within its unique state of consciousness The five brainwave states range from high arousal to deep dreamless sleep and are experienced by men, women and children of all ages, across all cultures Knowing about the various brainwaves enables us to understand what's happening in our brains as we engage in different activities, from studying for a quiz, to chilling with friends to enjoying deep restful sleep.

As you will see, counter to the high-speed pace of our culture today, faster is not always better when it comes to brain wave states.

BETA: WAKING STATE AND REASONING WAVE (14-40Hz)

GAMMA   SUPERCONSCIOUS
40-80 cycles per second

BETA   CONSCIOUS
13-39 cycles per second

ALPHA   SUBCONSCIOUS
8-13 cycles per second

THETA   SUPERCONSCIOUS
4-8 cycles per second

DELTA   DREAM STATE
0.5-4 cycles per second

Beta brain waves are associated with normal waking consciousness and a heightened state of alertness, critical thinking and logical reasoning. Beta brain waves are important for functioning throughout the day, as we face a myriad of choices from what to eat for lunch to what route we take home. When we engage in conversation, do homework, play video games or scan social media we are in Beta frequency.

While it is a necessary state, the Beta range can also lead to stress, anxiety, mental fatigue, burn out and agitation if we let our thinking mind spin out of control. It is here that we can encounter that negative inner critic that tends to dominate our attention if we're not careful. In our fast paced, productivity obsessed society, it's easy to see how most of us become consumed in the Beta state and succumb to the epidemic of stress related conditions that are commonplace today.

ALPHA: THE REST AND RELAXATION WAVE (7.5-14Hz)

At the Alpha brain wave level, we move into a comfortable state, with conscious awareness. This state is usually experienced with closed eyes, as we drift into an afternoon daydream or enter into a relaxed mindful state.

It is here where we step through the gateway of the subconscious mind, where we can reprogram and train our mind. The alpha state is where we can access our intuition—the ability to understand something without having to learn it intellectually—which is often inaccessible at faster frequencies. Intuition, a term derived from the Latin intueor, which means "to see", is what Steve Jobs called "more powerful than the intellect." Spending time in the alpha state also improves our imagination, memory, learning and concentration.

THETA: DEEP MINDFUL STATE (4-7.5HZ)

Theta brain waves are present during deep mindfulness practice as well as light sleep. Here we enter the realm of the subconscious mind, where our most deep-seated programs lie. This is the transitional state from waking (Alpha) to deep sleep (Delta) and from deep sleep back to waking. In a Theta state, we are able to reach profound states of stillness and present moment awareness, so it makes sense that we can touch boundless inspiration, creativity and insight in this frequency.

From 7Hz to 8Hz, at the Alpha-Theta juncture is where we access the creative power of our minds. It is the mental state where we can most readily create or recreate our own reality. At this frequency, you are aware of your surroundings however your body is in deep relaxation similarly experienced in deep Savasana, the resting pose in yoga. We effortlessly drop into this powerful state of quiet awareness in natural environments, so regularly spending time in the great outdoors is good for both your body and your mind.

DELTA: THE DEEP SLEEP WAVE (0.5-4HZ)

The Delta frequency is the slowest of the brain waves, which we experience in sound, dreamless sleep and very deep states of mindful awareness. Delta is said to be in the realm of our unconscious mind, also known to some as the Universal mind.

Deep sleep is an essential ingredient for wellbeing. It is where our cells regenerate, where we process our daily life experiences and where we restore our energy. You can imagine then, how detrimental it is on our minds and bodies to live with inadequate amounts of sleep. Research reveals that cell phones, iPads and laptops emit blue light which can prevent our brains from dropping into this deep state so it recommended to turn off devices, or at minimum, put them on airplane mode during sleep hours.

GAMMA: THE INSIGHT WAVE (ABOVE 40HZ)

This range is the most newly discovered and is the fastest frequency at above 40Hz. While little is known about this state of mind, early research shows Gamma waves are associated with rapid processing of information, bursts of insight and higher knowledge. Mindfulness practice, especially one that focuses on compassion increases gamma brainwaves, producing an ideal learning state, freedom from distract-ability, along with a sense of wholeness and well-being.

STUDENT REFLECTIONS

1) Can you see how this information on brain waves encourages you to create a life of balance by both challenging your brain to learn new things as well as giving it time to rest in open awareness?
2) What does your brain need more of right now to feel balanced, activity or rest?
3) Can you see the value of taking time out each day to rest your brain and drop the frequency with a mindfulness practice?

CARING FOR YOUR BRAIN

Your lifestyle diet is so much more than what you eat. It comprises everything you ingest; the shows you watch, the music you listen to, the content you read, even the company you hold. Therefore, if you are seeking success and happiness, be mindful of the things you consume, physically, mentally, emotionally and spiritually.

HIGH OCTANE BRAIN FOOD

Although your brain only makes up about 2% of your body weight (weighing in at about 3lbs), it uses a whopping 20% of your oxygen and caloric intake. Due to its energy demands and high fat content (about 60%), the human brain operates optimally on foods that are nutrient rich and high in healthy fats. Some examples of wholesome foods that are high in antioxidants that protect your brain from deterioration are: blueberries, turmeric, oranges, green tea and coffee (but remember this is the path of moderation) Other foods, such as fatty fish, nuts, seeds and eggs are considered optimal nutrition for brain development and memory.

STUDENT REFLECTION

1. If fruits, vegies, nuts and seafood are healthy choices for the brain, what foods cause deterioration of the brain, making mindfulness and focus even more challenging?
2. Research the effects that different foods and substances have on the brain, such as high sugar foods, energy drinks, deep fried foods, vegetable oils, drugs and alcohol.

YOUR BRAIN ON WATER

Not only does your brain require good nutrition, it also needs adequate hydration to function well. If you have trouble concentrating for any length of time, it might have something to do with your water intake. Research tells us that dehydration not only impairs our ability to pay attention but also negatively affects our short-term and long-term memory as well.

Over the course of a typical day, the longest period most of us go without food or fluid intake is the time we spend asleep. While we're enjoying deep slumber, the body sweats out toxins and each exhalation releases moisture from our lungs. Therefore, it makes good sense to 'break the fast' each morning with a tall glass of filtered, room temperature water. Adding a slice of lemon cleanses the colon and moves our bathroom routine in the right direction.

What's more, drinking water first thing in the morning kick starts your thirst instinct, which can become dulled if we let ourselves become dehydrated.

SLEEP—THE SECRET TO A HEALTHY BRAIN AND A SUCCESSFUL MINDFULNESS PRACTICE

The childhood years typically require about 10-12 hours of sleep a night, whereas adults require 7-9 hours Most people skimp on sleep throughout the week and spend the weekend attempting to catch up. A good night's sleep is an essential component of health and is necessary in order to sustain an effective mindfulness practice.

According to Frances E. Jenson, author of the Teenage Brain, sleep patterns change throughout our lives. She calls infants and children "larks" as they wake up early and go to sleep early. She then calls adolescents "owls" because they stay up late and sleep in in the morning. As we approach adulthood, we tend to revert back to the early to bed, early to rise pattern. The schedule we've culturally created for teens demands that they abide by our adult circadian rhythm, by rising early for school and work. But this early morning start apparently doesn't translate into an early night, as the teen brain tends to hold that part of the pattern What does that equate to? Exactly what we see in teens today: a chronically sleep deprived teenage population. The typical teenage body operates optimally on 9-10hrs of sleep per night and most teens today are getting a mere 6-8hrs, if they're lucky.

Jensen claims that sleep deprivation causes more than just physical fatigue. It can contribute to juvenile delinquency, criminal behavior, depression, obesity, high blood pressure and cardiovascular disease. [4] It also leads teens to consume more soft drinks, fried food, sweets and caffeine. Additionally, it leads to more screen time (which diminishes much needed melatonin), increased TV watching, less activity and higher rates of suicide.

Did you know that sleep integrates our learning from the day before, feeds our memory, improves athletic performance, helps us eat better and manage stress more effectively?

SIGNS OF SLEEP DEPRIVATION

- Fatigued throughout the day, especially mid afternoon
- Inability to concentrate clearly
- Dependence on a stimulant, such as caffeine, to successfully complete daily tasks
- Unexplained weight gain

---

[4] Frances E. Jensen, *The Teenage Brain*, (Colins, Jan 2015), 96

HELPFUL HINTS FOR GETTING A GOOD NIGHT SLEEP

- Avoid consuming heavy food past 7 pm.
- Step away from the screen in the evening to rest your optic nerve and restore melatonin.
- Remove all technological devices from your sleeping area and train your body to wake up naturally without an alarm. Set the intention to awake at the time your alarm goes off and soon your body will do it automatically. If using an alarm, have it turned on to uplifting, soft music to ease you into wakefulness.
- Feather your nest by creating a comforting and cozy sleeping environment.
- Be prepared and organized for the morning so you can relax into the moment.
- Right before you sleep, as you enter Theta wave state, is a great time to let your imagination wander. The last thing you think about is what you'll take into your dream world, so consciously create images or visions that will uplift your nighttime experience and bring you closer to your deepest dreams.
- Fill your nighttime routine with gentleness, beauty and *sattvic*/peaceful influences, such as reading by candle light, or gentle movement to soft music. Restorative asanas will help to deepen and slow your breathing, leading to a relaxed body state.
- Mindfulness calms and clears the mind of worry and overthinking. Affirm to yourself when worry arises, "This thought does not belong here".
- If your energy needs calming, sleepy time and camomile teas can be very effective.
- A darkened room is optimal for releasing melatonin, an essential hormone that repairs tissue and heals the body during sleep.
- Upon waking in the morning, take time to stretch, relax and count your blessings. Recall the deepest desires you have for your life and imagine stepping into them as you begin your day. Ask yourself whose life you can enhance by being present and through taking mindful action.
- If you're still having issues sleeping after implementing these suggestions, please consult with your doctor.

What else could you add to this list of suggestions? Is there anything you do that works in helping you sleep?

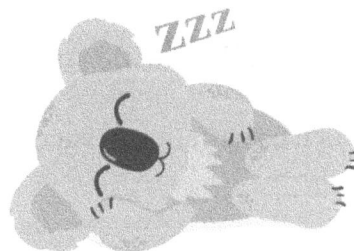

MINDFUL MEDICINE—A PHYSICIAN'S PERSPECTIVE

By: Dr. Maria Patriquin MD CCFP Family Physician and Mindfulness Specialist, Living Well Integrative Health Center, founder http://www.livingwellihc.ca/

Family medicine has a unique viewpoint derived from years of enduring relationships that span the lifecycle of a person and often generations of their families. It is a generalist practice, but great depth is formed through the sharing of life's ups and downs. Being privy to these deeply personal experiences has deepened my understanding of the events, environments, and genetic predispositions that influence how we develop into the people we become and the lives we live.

The seemingly simple practice of mindfulness is the basis on which I am able to form connections to patients, establishing a sense of safety and trust through active listening without judgment. This is particularly important for children and their families as judgment creates stigma and barriers to care. Being mindful enables me to process my own experience thereby enabling me to remain clear and capable of responding from a centered place. It also enables me to regulate my own emotional response while expressing empathy so that I can integrate information and creatively problem solve with my patients.

Without mindfulness we risk making more errors and projecting our perspective and expectations for health on our patients. Encounters that lack mindful awareness and compassionate exchange risk falling short of patients' needs and also risk causing people to make fear-based decisions rather than informed ones.

Children are the original mindfulness practitioners; therefore, we all began life with an innate ability to be mindful. With this natural inclination to be mindful, children derive pleasure easily, finding beauty in the unknown and familiar, sitting in awe and wonder of what to us might be simply a pile of dirt and sticks. This makes them perfectly poised for appreciation and gratitude. They have humor, laughing an average of 300 or more times a day. This speaks to their natural ability to be happy, make joy of anything and reduce stress or tension with a simple a hug. Children are naturally loving and affectionate.

The experiences and exposures we have in early life are formative and serve as the foundation of health from which we develop, learn and grow. How often do we hear the expression, "nature versus nurture"? The field of developmental psychology and neuroscience tell us that who we are, how we grow and evolve is our nature and "nature needs nurture!" We are social beings and the nurturing relationships we have early in life create neural, cognitive and emotional frameworks from which we form a sense of self and other.

Children are vulnerable and dependent on adults to nurture and protect their inherent qualities in an environment of safety, stability and stimulation. They need strong stable relationships and in doing so, children learn and grow in the healthiest of ways, reaching their maximal potential.

We live in a time where stress is the norm. Our society promotes fast foods, unhealthy sedentary lifestyles, detachment and isolation. Quick fixes and addictions are on the rise in our "on demand" culture, leading to more illness, band aid approaches, crisis-to-crisis coping that inevitably causes more stress. Every single child I counsel, from age 5 to 18, when asked,

"If you could change one thing to make your life better, what would it be?" have answered, "I wish my parent/s were less stressed or depressed." Every single one.

Adverse childhood experiences (ACEs) are events that can have potentially traumatic, negative, lasting effects on health and well-being. These experiences range from physical, emotional, or sexual abuse to parental divorce, parental mental illness, witnessing domestic violence, family dysfunction and neglect. ACEs encompass bullying, discrimination (due to race, ethnicity, sexual orientation, disability or culture) medical trauma, deportation and migration, involvement with foster care, death of a parent, living in an unsafe neighborhood and witnessing community violence, however, this is not an exhaustive list.

Research has repeatedly demonstrated that two thirds of the population have had at least one ACE. 40% have two or more and 12-15 % have more than four ACEs. ACEs cluster and have a strong cumulative effect on health and wellbeing throughout the lifespan, leading to exponentially higher risk of learning, behavioral, social and health problems. Not exclusively these include obesity, some cancers, heart, liver and lung disease, depression, substance abuse and poor academic achievement. Those with higher ACE scores are at increased risk for high risk sexual behaviors including early sexual activity, teen pregnancy, sexually transmitted disease and intimate partner violence. Those with an ACE score of four are twice as likely to be smokers and seven times more likely to be alcoholic. An ACE score of four increases the risk of COPD by 400 percent and attempted suicide by 1200 percent. Those with an ACE score of six or higher are at risk of their lifespan being shortened by as much as twenty years.

In today's world, our ACEs are high. Over a million Canadian children are affected by mental health issues and less than 20% will receive the care they require. After accidents, suicide is the second leading cause of death. Canada is one of five countries with the highest rates of teen suicide. One in four children live in poverty, the highest rates are in Manitoba and the Maritime provinces. One in ten children have food insecurity. 25% of children will experience developmental vulnerability which means that their readiness and ability to learn is compromised before they even enter school. Canadian children are less physically active than other countries and 25% are obese. We are clearly falling short of meeting the physical, cognitive and emotional needs of children in Canada.

Through a mindful, compassionate lens, children become humans struggling to imperfectly communicate their needs in a stressful adult-centric, hurried world. It is critical that children have a voice and are heard otherwise they risk thinking "they are the problem" rather than seeing they "have a problem". In an atmosphere of safety and compassion, children can courageously share deep fears, depressive thoughts, worry, and anxiety. They can express grief, anger, reveal substance use, abuse, stress, suicidal tendencies and confusion. Creating a safe space for children to speak up helps them to integrate their life experiences.

When we hold children's vulnerability with respect and care, they begin to believe they can too. With repeated practice, they develop skills and form relationships based on self-respect, self-compassion. Mindful, compassionate exchanges empower children to realize their worth and value, and with that awareness, they can harness their strengths and thrive.

For six years now, I have led stress reduction groups. After eight weeks, a roomful of strangers foster deep and lasting connections through a shared sense of humanity. I teach mindfulness techniques that calm the sympathetic nervous system, that teach us how to hold intense feelings and to use cognitive strategies to work with negative thoughts. Participants learn that empathy and compassion for oneself and others are at the heart of health and healing. When asked if they could change just one thing, the majority of participants respond, "I wish I learned this as a child."

It is time to consider a new curriculum for care, education and parenting. In order for us to evolve as a species, we must harness our innate wisdom. We live in a knowledge economy, yet only we can impart personal values, the very ones we complain children are lacking. Let's consider a new curriculum based on mindfulness, that emphasizes and nurtures care, character, conscience, communication, conciliation, courage, contribution, collaboration and compassion.

Childhood is a precious short time. We were once children and that child remains within. The way we treat ourselves and each other becomes the voice with which we parent, teach and lead. How we treat and teach children becomes their inner voice. Through an awareness of mindfulness, compassion and kindness, we can more fully understand our children, and thus help to instill within them a sense of wholeness, worth and value. My hope is that we become part of a larger conversation that leads to meaningful improvements in the lives of children and the adults they will become.

How do I Feel: The Interoception & Mindfulness Connection

By: Kelly Mahler, author of Interoception: the eighth sensory system.
https://www.mahlerautism.com/interoception

How do you know when you feel sleepy? Perhaps it is because you notice heavy feeling eyes, a fuzzy brain or sluggish muscles. How do you know when you feel stressed? Maybe it is because you notice tense muscles, a pounding head, upset stomach or sweaty palms. How do you know when you feel calm? Perhaps it is because you notice that your muscles are loose, head is clear, stomach is content or palms are dry. In all of these cases, you use these important clues coming from your body to help you determine your current emotion in any given moment. You are able to experience these body clues with the help of a little-known, but extremely important sense called interoception.

What is Interoception?

Interoception is a sense - similar to vision, touch and hearing - only rather than collecting sensory information from the world around you, outside of your body, interoception collects sensory information from the inside of your body. Interoception collects this information from a variety of internal body areas including your heart, stomach, bladder, intestines, muscles, skin, bones, and even eyes. This information is sent to the brain where it is used to figure out how these body areas feel. For example, information collected from the stomach will let you know how your stomach feels: does it feel empty, heavy, gassy, nauseous, tingly or something else? The specific way your stomach feels provides you with clues to your current emotion: are you hungry, full, sick, nervous and so forth? Interoception is constantly working behind the scenes, gathering information in order to let you clearly experience a wide variety of emotions including: hunger, fullness, thirst, illness, pain, need for bathroom, sexual arousal, relaxation, anger, anxiety, joy, or even physical exhaustion.

Therefore, interoception provides you with information about the internal condition of your body, which in turn informs your emotions, and allows you to answer the question, "How do I feel?"

The Importance of Listening to Your Body

Those individuals that are more aware of the interoception feelings within their body are described as having good levels of Interoceptive Awareness (IA). This ability to both: (a) notice internal body signals and (b) give meaning to the internal signals. For example, you may notice a dry feeling in your mouth and throat and know that it means you are thirsty. Or you may notice shakiness in your muscles, a quivering stomach and faster heart and know that it means that you are nervous. Interoceptive awareness plays the starring role in this ability to notice and interpret the internal feelings of the body.

The degree in which we are aware of signals from within our body varies from person to person. Research has found that people with good awareness of their internal body signals are more mindful of their emotions and are able to control and adjust their emotions with greater levels of success. This is because people with good levels of IA are able to clearly notice and understand body clues which urges them into healthy actions. For example, if you clearly notice sensations of fullness you are urged to stop eating. Or if you clearly notice small levels of stress building you are urged to use a strategy to decompress before the stress gets too intense. On the opposite end, some people have lower levels of IA and may not detect certain body signals at all, or at least not until the body signals are very, very intense. This can make quickly recognizing and managing emotions very difficult. Nick, a 17-year old high school student, shares "Many times, I don't notice that I am getting angry until I am exploding with anger. By then it is too late. There is very little I can do to get control."

WHAT'S MINDFULNESS GOT TO DO WITH IT?

Research has found that mindfulness is one of the most effective methods of enhancing IA. In fact the use of certain mindfulness exercises can improve your awareness in as little as 8 weeks. Paying attention to your body in a certain way without judgement, which is a hallmark of mindfulness, helps you to focus on the body signals occurring in your body at the present moment By making it a habit to become more aware of your interoceptive body signals, you can gain better insight into your body and emotions, thus ultimately improving your control over the way you feel.

PRACTICE MAKES PERFECT

When practicing mindfulness with the specific goal of maximizing IA, a few things are helpful to keep in mind.

1. Practice noticing body signals during neutral or positive feeling emotions first. This is a hallmark of interoception treatment in the trauma field but is good practice for all. Creating opportunities to notice comfortable feeling body signals, begins the mindfulness journey from a place of openness and positivity.

2. Link comfortable body signals to the cause. Once you are mindful of comfortable feeling body signals, determine the cause of the comfortable feelings (e.g. maybe it is the quiet song playing in the background, or perhaps it is a certain person that you are sitting nearby, or maybe it is the breathing pattern that you are using). This helps to build individualized, in-the-moment connections with those experiences that make you feel good. These concrete connections can help you develop a wider variety of feel-good, self-care strategies.

3. All body signals are important: there are no 'good' or 'bad' body signals. Once you gradually begin noticing certain body signals that might not feel quite as comfortable (e.g. growling stomach, full bladder, tense muscles), notice them from a place of non-judgement. All body signals are important. Noticing the way your body can feel can be source of empowerment, as it gives you insight and control over the way you feel. Do

you have a quickly approaching deadline and you notice a fast heart, tight chest and shaky muscles? These body signals inform your emotion: that you are feeling stressed. It can be helpful to accept these body signals as a great sign that your body is gearing up to help you meet the deadline In this case, stress will be a driving force to keep you motivated towards the goal (deadline). Keep the stress at a helpful level by using self-care strategies learned in tip 2.

4. Keep in mind that each person's body-emotion connections are very different. In other words, we each feel emotions differently. What your body feels like when you are relaxed will be different than what another person's body feels like when they are relaxed. Over time, continually linking the body signals noticed during mindful moments to a specific emotion, can give concrete meaning to an emotion. The emotion becomes more than just a word, it becomes rooted in a concrete collection of body signals that is self-discovered through mindfulness practice.

In summary, interoception is a little known, but very important sense. It is widely studied in fields such as neuroscience and medicine but is only very recently is making the way into practical application in daily life. Interoception allows us to notice and understand signals coming from within our body and is at the base of the body-emotion connection. Mindfulness, which can teach us to better listen to our body, is an evidenced-based method for developing good levels of interoceptive awareness. Research indicates that good awareness of our interoception body signals is important for many different aspects of life including emotional self-awareness, emotional control and emotional well-being. Therefore, in addition to countless other benefits of mindfulness practice, or living mindfully, building awareness of interoception body signals is near the top of the list.

COMPLEMENTARY MINDFUL MOVEMENT PRACTICE

If time allows, proceed through 'Movement Flow for Emotional Ease' or the 'Art Therapy Movement Class' with the intention of maintaining this centered, grounded focus.

ZONES OF REGULATION

By Leah Kuypers, author of The Zones of Regulation,
http://www.zonesofregulation.com/index.html

WHAT IS SELF-REGULATION?

Self-regulation can go by many names, such as "self-control," "self-management," "anger control," and "impulse control." These terms all describe people's ability to adjust their level of alertness and how they display their emotions through their behavior to attain goals in socially adaptive ways (Bronson, 2001). In other words, self-regulation is the ability to do what needs to be done to be in the optimal state for the given situation. This includes regulating one's sensory needs, emotions, and impulses to meet the demands of the environment, reach one's goals, and behave in a socially appropriate way. For example, given a stressful or frustrating experience, a person who can self-regulate well is able to remain calm and organized to successfully negotiate the event. If a person who struggles with self-regulation encounters the same frustrating experience, he or she will have difficulty coping and display maladaptive behaviors. To successfully self-regulate, three critical neurological components need be integrated: sensory processing, executive functioning, and emotional regulation.

SENSORY PROCESSING

The first neurological component, sensory processing, describes how you make sense of the information perceived by your sensory receptors (the nerve endings that respond to stimuli) as well as how you organize and integrate the information so that you can act upon it in a purposeful way. For example, the sound of a fire alarm is first perceived by your ear. That information is then relayed to your brain to be interpreted-in this case, as a fire alarm going off. You then determine if this is a stimulus you need to attend to or filter out. (Most likely, action is needed if a fire alarm goes off, but often you don't act when someone else's car alarm goes off because you are so used to hearing that sound.) If you determine that action is needed, your body is organized so it can purposefully respond, such as to calmly walk out of the building.

Sensory processing also includes modulating the amount of sensory input you receive so that you don't become overwhelmed by too much of a stimulus. For instance, many younger children love all of the spinning rides at a carnival and can ride on them repeatedly without becoming dizzy. Adults tend to avoid rides such as the Tilt-a-Whirl so they don't become sick or nauseated by the spinning; they know they need to modulate that kind of stimulus. Another example of modulating sensory input is that many people often unconsciously shut off their radio if they are driving a car and hit traffic. By reducing one sensation (the sound from the radio), they are better able to focus on the more important visual information that they need to process (the road and traffic) and feel more in control.

Sensory processing disorder, also called sensory integration dysfunction, first described by occupational therapist A. Jean Ayres in the 1970s, refers to a person having difficulties with receiving sensory information, processing it, and/or responding to it. Sensory input includes the following types of information: visual, auditory (hearing), tactile (touch), olfactory (smell), gustatory (taste), vestibular (movement and body's relationship to gravity), and proprioception (body awareness).

Difficulties in regulation can result from people not being able to filter out extraneous stimuli or being overly sensitive to small amounts of a sensation that most others don't find offensive or notice (known as being hyper-responsive). For example, a student in the classroom has the relevant stimuli they need to process (e.g., the teacher talking, notes on the board) but may be overwhelmed by all the background sensory information that they have difficulty filtering out (e.g., the tags on their clothing itching, noise in the hallway, excessive artwork/ visuals hung in the classroom, smell coming from the lunchroom), resulting in the student appearing distracted, irritated, and restless. In contrast, some people seek out intense input in one or more of their senses to feel just right. This is known as being hypo-responsive to that input and can be very disruptive to others if the sensory seeking is not done in a purposeful and meaningful way. For example, some students need additional movement and deep pressure to their bodies to feel focused and ready to learn and may find ways to experience the movement and deep pressure that is perceived by others as inappropriate (e.g., rolling around on the carpet during circle time, getting out of their chair frequently, bumping into others, hanging upside down from their chair). Giving such students meaningful opportunities throughout the day to experience additional movement, heavy work, and deep pressure (e.g., running a note to the office, pushing the ball cart out to recess, erasing the board, passing out papers) will help those students get the sensory input they need to organize their nervous system and be attentive. Our ability to self-regulate depends largely upon how well our brain organizes the information our sensory system provides. We want to be able to integrate the information to meet a purpose. For example, as we hear someone talking, we want to be able to respond with appropriate speech or other communication. If we see a ball being thrown toward us, we want to be able to respond with our arms outstretched to catch it. At other times, we will want to ignore sensory information to prevent becoming over-whelmed or distracted. The Zones of Regulation addresses sensory processing by helping students understand what supports they need to feel regulated.

EXECUTIVE FUNCTIONING

The next critical neurological component of self-regulation is executive functioning, which is a general term that describes the cognitive processes involved in the conscious control of thoughts and actions. Executive functioning can be compared to a command or control center in our brains that oversees actions and mental operations. Our ability to self-regulate depends on the effectiveness of these functions. Numerous mental operations fall under executive functioning, but some that are influential to the ability to self-regulate are: attention shifting (attending to two or more activities simultaneously, such as taking notes while listening to a lecture), working memory (updating and purging "files" in the brain with new information), internalization of speech (self-talk): flexible thinking (considering multiple options), planning (organizing actions and executing a plan in order to reach desired goals) and inhibition (impulse control). When these cognitive processes function adequately, students are better equipped to complete the problem solving necessary to overcome the hurdles they meet.

Various teaching strategies, including The Zones, can be used to help students gain skills in consciously mediating their actions, which in turn leads to increased control and problem-solving abilities.

CONTROLLING EMOTIONS

The third critical component of self-regulation is the ability to control emotions. Emotional regulation can be defined as processes that are responsible for controlling your emotional reactions in order to meet your goal. This includes monitoring, evaluating, and modifying the intensity and timing of your emotional response. Aristotle put it best, "Anyone can become angry, that is easy...but to be angry with the right person, to the right degree, at the right time, for the right purpose, and in the right way...this is not easy." As described in Russell Barkley's research (an internationally recognized authority on attention deficit hyperactive disorder), emotions are automatically triggered in response to events. However, cognitive elements, such as having objectivity (determining the size of the problem), motivation, and understanding others' perspectives are used in regulating the emotion. Students who struggle with these skills have a more difficult time regulating their emotions. These are skills that The Zones of Regulation curriculum addresses to help students become successful in self-regulation.

All three of these neurological components-sensory processing, executive functioning, and emotional regulation-depend on one another. If one of these components does not function adequately, the person's ability to self-regulate will be diminished-so it is important to look at all three This is a brief overview of self-regulation processes. If you'd like to learn more, you can refer to the literature review available at www.ZonesOfRegulation.com.

WHAT ARE THE ZONES OF REGULATION?

The Zones of Regulation is a conceptual framework used to teach students self-regulation. Creating this type of system to categorize the complex feelings and states students experience improves their ability to recognize and communicate how they are feeling in a safe, non-judgmental way. It also allows students to tap into strategies or tools to help them move between zones. The Zones of Regulation categorizes states of alertness and emotions into four colored zones

The Blue Zone

Used to describe low states of alertness, such as when one feels sad, tired, sick, or bored. This is when one's body and/or brain is moving slowly or sluggishly.

The Green Zone

Used to describe a regulated state of alertness. A person may be described as calm, happy, focused, or content when in the Green Zone. This is the zone students generally need to be in for schoolwork and for being social. Being in the Green Zone shows control.

The Yellow Zone

Also used to describe a heightened state of alertness; however, a person has some control when in the Yellow Zone. A person may be experiencing stress, frustration, anxiety, excitement, silliness, nervousness, confusion, and many more slightly elevated emotions and states when in the Yellow Zone (such as wiggly, squirmy, or sensory seeking). The Yellow Zone is starting to lose some control.

The Red Zone

Used to describe extremely heightened states of alertness or very intense feelings. A person may be experiencing anger, rage, explosive behavior, panic, or terror when in the Red Zone. Being in the Red Zone can best be explained by not being in control of one's body.

The zones can be compared to a stoplight or traffic signs. When given a green light (in the Green Zone), one is "good to go." A yellow light or caution sign means slow down or take warning, which applies to the Yellow Zone. A red light or stop sign means stop; when a person is in the Red Zone, he or she needs to stop and regain control. The Blue Zone can be compared to a blue rest area where you pull over when you're tired and need to recharge.

It is important to note and reiterate to students that everyone experiences all of the zones at one time or another; the Red and Yellow Zones are not the " bad" or "naughty" zones. Make sure not to tell a student one zone is good and another is bad. Rather, you will teach students to figure out what zone is expected in given circumstances. If their zone doesn't match the environmental demands and the zones of others around them, you will be teaching strategies to assist them in moving to the expected zone. The Zones of Regulation is intended to be neutral and not project judgment when helping students recognize their levels of alertness and feelings.

It is easy to point out to students when they are in the Red and Yellow Zones. However, if the different colored zones are used only to indicate to students when they are not doing what is expected, they will surely become averse to practicing it. Be sure you provide positive reinforcement when they are in the Green Zone as well as when they make efforts to remain in the Green Zone when encountering situations that lead them to less regulated states. When they are in a zone, a simple acknowledgement or labeling of that zone will be helpful in recognizing when they are there.

MINDFULNESS AND AUTISM

By: Catherine Rahey, M.Ed, B.ED, co-author of Yoga for Autism

There is an emerging body of research that's evaluating the effectiveness of mindfulness interventions for reducing anxiety, stress, aggression, dysregulation, depression and rumination in individuals with Autism Spectrum Disorder (ASD) The studies are also investigating whether these mindfulness interventions produce a positive affect on psychological well-being in individuals with ASD, and the results indicating that they receive positive benefits if Mindfulness interventions are implemented systemically with consistency and dedication.

These Mindfulness based programs focus on training participants to pay attention to the present moment, on purpose and with a non-judgmental, openhearted, and curious attitude (Kabat-Zinn 1994). They train enhanced attention and awareness of experiences such as senses, bodily sensations, thoughts and feelings.

Autism Spectrum Disorder (ASD) is characterized by difficulties in social communication and interaction, while demonstrating repetitive and restrictive behaviour patterns, interests, or activities (American Psychiatric Association 2013) There is much research that implies individuals with ASD have significant deficits in the area of Interoception – the sensory system that gives us information regarding the internal condition of our body (Craig 2002; Mahler 2016).

Individuals with ASD often lack the ability to:

- recognize the bodily sensation
- give meaning to the sensation (body state or emotion)
- take appropriate action that provides a solution

These can be key factors in the high anxiety, stress and aggression levels in individuals with ASD Mindfulness practices can be very helpful in understanding one's internal bodily state which may result in a more focused, calm and attentive frame of mind for individuals with ASD.

As an Autism Consultant with thirty-five years' experience, I have found that teaching Interoception through mindfulness practices is the first step in fostering concentration and stress reduction, as well as for managing dysregulated behaviour towards unknown situations.

CENTRAL COHERENCE SYSTEM

Some individuals with ASD have the ability to see the details of a situation but may have difficulty seeing the whole picture. The ability to do both would suggest a strong "central coherence system" With mindfulness practice we are able to teach students how to shift their focus from the narrow details to the whole situation, depending upon the need, thereby improving their central coherence. Rather than paying excessive attention to details that consume their attention unnecessarily, participants learn to view both internal and external experiences as passing events in a wider field of awareness (Kabat-Zinn 1994; Segal et al. 2012). With proper training and diligent practice, the underlying neurocognitive needs may improve.

Here are a few strategies to Support Mindfulness practices to Improve Central Coherence.

Note: we should always include the parents/guardians in the education, so they can reinforce the strategies at home.

1. There are three types of social narratives that provide direct instruction of social situations for individuals with autism. Each strategy provides a visual cue and desired social responses. The content should match the individual's needs and take their perspective into consideration.

    a. A Social Story - "A Social Story accurately describes a context, skill, achievement, or concept according to 10 defining criteria. These criteria guide story research, development, and implementation to ensure an overall patient and supportive quality, and a format, "voice", content, and learning experience that is descriptive, meaningful, and physically, socially, and emotionally safe for the child, adolescent, or adult with autism. "(Carol Gray 2018).

    b. A Comic Strip Conversation – A comic strip conversation uses simple drawings to visually outline a conversation between two or more people who may be reporting the past, describing the present or planning for the future. These drawings serve to illustrate ongoing communication and to provide additional support to individuals who struggle to understand the quick exchange of information that occurs in social situations. Comic strip conversations are based on the belief that visual supports may improve the understanding and comprehension of social situations (Gray, 1994).

    c. Power Cards – this is a strategy that involves including special interests with visual aids to teach and reinforce skills to individuals with Autism Spectrum Disorders. By using their special interest, the individual is motivated to use the strategy presented in the scenario and on the Power Card.(Elisa Gagnon)

2. Pre-Teach the practice through created structures, visual systems and work systems. Pre-Teach, Teach and Re-teach. Practice, practice, practice.

3. Visualization and Mindfulness practices.

4. Nature, environmental exploration where students visually see the big picture and shift to the details allowing for practice of narrowing and widening the experience. This should be in an environment that is calm and quiet like the beach or a forest.

5. Use visuals and decrease the oral language instruction.

6. Practice interoception and yoga practices such as the Body Scan, focusing on one part of the body at a time. Start with the outer body parts first and then proceed towards the internal organs. Always start with the easiest body part and work towards the more difficult. Take your time and go deep with the teaching of each body part.

EXECUTIVE FUNCTIONING

Many individuals with ASD may also have deficits with regards to executive functioning. It is thought this is one of the core areas of deficits for many individuals with various developmental complex needs.

Executive functioning includes skills such as

1. organizing
2. planning
3. attention to task
4. sustaining attention
5. responding appropriately to the environment

Executive Functioning could be improved through mindfulness as it trains a person to control focused attention, to flexibly shift attention, to reflect on one's experiences, and to notice one's automatic impulses which enables one to respond with awareness instead of reacting impulsively (Zelazo and Lyons 2012).

Many executive function capacities are connected to mindfulness training. More specifically, research has suggested that practicing for extended periods of time and even for shortened lengths of time can have lasting positive effects on participants' attentional capacities, memories, moods, alertness and levels of anxiety or depression This is supported in a study that reported that people who practiced mindfulness for only four days improved their moods, verbal fluencies, visual coding and working memories (Ziedan, Johnson, Diamond, David & Goolkasian, 2010).

Here are a few strategies to support Mindfulness practices for Executive Functioning
1. Begin with Breathing Exercises.
2. Mindful movements.
3. Guided visualizations, which must be pre-taught and accompanied by visual supports.
4. Mindful minute exercises incorporating yoga movements.
5. Body Awareness and Focus (Interoception activities- Kelly Mahler).
6. Yoga and Autism, Circle of Light – Jenny Kierstead and Catherine Rahey.
7. Visual Structures, Visual Systems and Visual Boundaries.

Instead of being caught up in negative thoughts, individuals can be taught to practice becoming more aware of the connection between bodily sensations, feelings, and thoughts. This training can reduce heightened levels of stress, emotional, and behavioural concerns as well as improve social communication and interaction with others. Being able to understand and pay more attention to social interactions, instead of getting distracted by ruminating thoughts or sounds in the environment can lead to better self-awareness and a greater ability to attend to others. Through mindfulness practice, one becomes more aware of their emotions, leading to a better understanding of emotional processes and may improve the ability to understand others' emotions. Also, mindfulness may lead to increased awareness of the effect of one's own behaviors on others (Block-Lerner et al. 2007; Sequeira and Ahmed 2012).

In conclusion, Mindfulness-based programs help improve individuals with autism's ability to cope, understand and navigate the various social interactions and nuisances they will inevitably encounter throughout their day. Through practice, individuals can learn to relate to themselves and others with less judgment and more curiosity and compassion.

TRAUMA-SENSITIVE MINDFULNESS

By: David A. Treleaven, author of Trauma-Sensitive Mindfulness,
https://www.davidtreleaven.com

Mindfulness can enhance present-moment awareness, increase our self-compassion, and enhance our ability to self, regulate But mindfulness can also generate problems for people struggling with traumatic stress When we ask someone with trauma to pay close, sustained attention to their internal world, we invite them into contact with traumatic stimuli--thoughts, images, memories, and physical sensations that may relate to a traumatic event. As my friend experienced, this can aggravate and intensify symptoms of traumatic stress, in some cases even lead to re-traumatization--a relapse into an intensely traumatized state.

This raises crucial questions for those of us offering mindfulness instruction. What is our responsibility to people experiencing trauma? Is a certain amount of pain to be expected in practice? How can we know when a survivor should or shouldn't be practicing? And how can we grasp our own limitations in understanding other people's experiences of trauma, as a way to best support them?

In sum, how can we offer mindfulness in a trauma sensitive way?

Trauma-sensitive, or trauma-informed, practice means that we have a basic understanding of trauma in the context of our work. A trauma, informed physician can ask a patient's permission before touching them, for example. Or a trauma-informed school counselor might ask a student whether they want the door open or closed during a session and inquire about a comfortable sitting distance. With trauma-informed mindfulness, we apply this concept to mindfulness instruction. We commit to recognizing trauma, responding to it skillfully, and taking pre-emptive steps to ensure that people aren't retraumatizing themselves under our guidance.

The need for trauma-sensitive mindfulness is a reflection of both odds and statistics. Over the past decade, mindfulness has exploded in popularity It is now being offered in a wide range of secular environments, including elementary and high schools, corporations, and hospitals. Any number of workshops, retreats, conferences, seminars, and institutes offer mindfulness instruction. Books and articles on the subject have flooded the marketplace At the same time, the prevalence of trauma is extraordinarily high. The majority of us will be exposed to at least some type of traumatic event in our lifetime, and some of us will develop debilitating symptoms in its aftermath. If we're targeted by systemic oppression -as someone who is poor or working class, disabled, a person of color, transgender, or a woman-we face a greater likelihood of experiencing interpersonal trauma over the course of our lives, and live inside of traumatic conditions every day.

What this means is that in any environment where mindfulness is being practiced, there's a high likelihood that someone will be struggling with traumatic stress. From a student who witnessed domestic violence to an elderly person who recently lost their partner in a fall, trauma will often be present. And while not everyone who has experienced trauma will have an adverse response to mindfulness, we need to be prepared for this possibility.

GUIDELINES FOR TRAUMA INFORMED MINDFULNESS TEACHING

Before asking our students or clients to sit down and be present to all the sensations in their bodies and become aware of the stream of thoughts running through their minds, it's essential to know a little bit about trauma. Trauma is defined by the American Psychological Association (APA) as the emotional response someone has to an extremely distressing event. Signs of trauma can occur immediately after an event or days or even months later. A person who has incurred trauma may withdraw from social situations, or become anxious, depressed, irritable or moody. If the traumatic event is not fully integrated and understood, a person may develop PTSD (post-traumatic stress disorder).

Students who have difficulty sitting still or concentrating may well have attention deficits, but there is also a chance they may be suffering from PTSD and simply attempting to manage or avoid painful sensations. PTSD therefore, requires its own treatment protocol, not a typical mindfulness practice.

Here are a few suggestions for leading a mindfulness class with an awareness of trauma

1. External anchors: In mindfulness there is a lot of emphasis placed on cultivating interoception, through practices like the Body Scan, that hone our ability to read and understand the internal messages of the body. Trauma survivors, however, may find this inward focus overwhelming, and therefore can begin with exteroceptive awareness, becoming present to external anchors through the senses, such as sights, sounds or sensations. Practices such as Awakening the Senses in the mindfulness section and the Five Finger Practice in the movement section both support this exteroceptive awareness.

2. Personal autonomy: since trauma survivors needs are varied and unique, encourage all students to claim responsibility for their needs by making choices that invoke safety such as sitting instead of lying down or keeping eyes slightly open instead of closing them during mindful practices. Encourage them to also be aware of triggering postures and to choose 'body shapes' that feel safe (note that words such as 'postures' or 'positions' may be trigger words).

3. Challenge by choice: in terms of participation, always affirm that they have choice with regards to their degree of involvement.

4. Compassion: despite the fact that nobody chooses to be traumatized, a survivor may harbour shame about their situation and their mental state. One of the most powerful remedies for shame is compassion. Teachers of mindfulness can offer compassion to all students and also encourage students to be gentle and compassionate with themselves.

5. Shared humanity: given that about 90% of people experience a traumatic event in their lives, reassuring students that they are not alone can help comfort and ease the shame that often accompanies trauma.

6. Respect your growing edge: encourage students to sit quietly during mindfulness practice, but also give them permission to honor their growing edge by shifting around if they need to. Some students may even need to leave the room initially and return as they're ready. Be aware that the instinct to avoid unpleasant memories or sensations may be an important coping mechanism but it may also be preventing a person from

moving forward in his/her life.

7. Gradual exposure: consider doing shorter practices at a time, over an extended period of time instead of suddenly immersing your students in lengthy practices right away.

8. Invite vs demand: be mindful about the wording and tone of your instructions, using invitatory language which implies choice, instead of demanding language which implies control.

9. Physical and emotional boundaries: create well defined physical boundaries, such as the hoola hoop activity or the use of a yoga mat. Read the Mindful Classroom Agreement to clarify what it means to behave respectfully and have all students agree to it.

10. Set up support: whenever we introduce practices that draw awareness to our thoughts, sensations or emotions, it is wise to be prepared with a list of professionals skilled in dealing with trauma so that students can augment their mindfulness practice with personalized treatment if or when needed.

MINDFUL PRACTICES FOR SELF-REGULATION

Practice is a term used a lot in most mindfulness resources because it is a health promoting strategy that requires intentional, consistent effort (also known as practice☺) One of the benefits from mindful practices is self-regulation. When we are able to regulate our behavior, we are able to act in a way that is congruent with our deepest values. If we struggle to regulate our behavior, we run risk of violating our values which can lead to destructive emotions such as guilt, shame, frustration, anxiety, all of which are emotions that compromise our wellbeing. For example, if a person values respect but acts in a way that diminishes another's self-esteem, he may be riddled with shame after the encounter. By improving self-regulation, we can more readily conduct ourselves in ways that align with our values, fostering a sense of inner harmony and integrity.

When we are able to regulate our emotions, we're capable of adjusting our inner emotional environment, (like calming ourselves when we feel triggered or reassuring ourselves when we feel disappointed) without external intervention. Therefore, developing self-regulation can be very empowering and cultivate confidence. It must be noted however, that emotional regulation is a challenging feat to achieve on our own, which speaks to the importance of having a supportive social network.

The following are short, effective techniques that nurture self-regulation by helping to focus the mind, balance emotions and calm the body. Additionally, each of the following exercises include the three basic components of any mindfulness practice

1. The person who is practicing
2. The technique being applied
3. The object of concentration or tool used to maintain mindful awareness.

Before we jump in, here are a few details for teachers to consider.

CREATING A CALM, MINDFUL ENVIRONMENT

Regardless of the grade you teach or the type of work you do, mindfulness can infiltrate any learning environment and complement every lesson.

Within your work space, it is suggested to allocate a spot for mindfulness practice. The children can decide on a name for it, whether it's the 'Calming Corner', the space for a 'Mindful Moment', or a place for a 'Time-in' (versus a time out). You could also couple this space with the concept of a sensory room, where children can go to restore emotional balance and be still. Invite your students to contribute to the creation of this space, by adding cozy or weighted blankets, soft cushions or stuffies, aromatherapy, calming music etc.

As a collective, you can take time to create a list of guidelines for the treatment of the space, such as

- No food or drink,
- No technology (except for the purpose of music)
- Minimal conversation or whispers only
- Depending on the size of the space, limit the number of people who utilize the space at a time

- Clean up before you leave

Students or clients are also invited to create a special place in their own lives for self-reflective, mindfulness work. Whether it's a corner table in the bedroom or a whole room in their house, they can work with what they have and design it to reflect their deepest values and highest visions. They can add inspiring images and symbolic items like stones, shells or candles that help to create a nurturing environment of goodness and peace.

PERSONAL SAFETY

In terms of personal space, having a clear defined boundary will be important for students whose personal safety has been compromised. Using a hoola hoop, a yoga mat or even a chair as a visual boundary can help to clarify students' personal space, for themselves and other students. See Mindful Games section for more on the hoola hoop.

RITUAL

One of the most powerful ways we can leverage the amazing results of mindfulness is to practice the simple art of ritual. Ritual is the act of doing something routinely with mindful awareness, while holding the intention of connecting with our true self. Rituals help to release old, outmoded habits, and invoke ways of being that are more aligned with our deepest desires. Ritual can become a daily reminder of our desire to become a more peaceful, self-assured person in the world.

The mind and body respond well to consistency; therefore, it is recommended to set aside the same time in the same place each day to do your mindfulness practice. Your health and wellbeing are worthy of this time, even if it's just five minutes each day. It is advised to aim for twenty minutes a day since it can take time to settle down and immerse oneself into the practice.

PRACTICES FOR REGULATING THE MIND

PRESENT MOMENT ANCHORS

So much of the distress we experience in any given moment stems from the memory of a stressful event in the past and the fear that our future will involve more of what we've already endured. Intentionally drawing our minds into the present moment can help us see the situation more clearly for what it is. A simple way of drawing the mind away from a stressful past event is to first engage 1:2 ratio breathing, and then begin focusing on an object within our current environment, using it as a present moment anchor for your mind. Ideally, choose an item that stimulates multiple senses, such as a bird that can be seen and heard, or a soft pillow that can be felt and seen or warm tea that can be smelled, tasted and felt.

PEAK POSITIVITY

Knowing that our minds instinctively favor negativity that leads us down the rabbit hold of dark, depressing thought patterns, we can use our awareness to shift gears when we notice ourselves sliding into its abyss As our mindfulness practice develops, we'll become more skillful at recognizing when we've lost our mind to negative or fatalistic thinking. With that awareness, we can press the pause button on the stream of thoughts and swap the negative for a more constructive thought. In order for us to reach our peak positivity potential, it is recommended that for each negative, destructive thought it takes a counter force of three positive, supportive thoughts to change the pattern. For example, the next time you look in the mirror and notice a criticism arise, shift your perspective to three encouraging, positive qualities and let your mind rest on these positives for a few minutes. Positivity leads to gratitude and gratitude leads to whole-heartedness. When you live in a whole-hearted way, you frequently experience magical moments, where your heart fills with a sense of wonder, joy and connection.

FALLING UP

When something doesn't go as planned, most people mope around and look for more signs that they're bad luck is on a roll. Successful people, however, train themselves to use their failures and disappointments as fuel for their revival. When they fall down, they stand up, brush themselves off, learn from their mistakes and move on with even greater determination. This is resilience. In order to fall UP, we must train ourselves to expect to be delighted by supportive and positive surprises. Assuming an optimistic attitude buffers the effects of stress and helps us become more resilient, leading to bounce-back moments. Although it's not a natural instinct to look for the good, we can all benefit from assuming the faith that everything on our path is, in one way or another, helping us to fall UP into our best life.

THINK BIG PICTURE

The next time you catch yourself becoming narrow focused, making a small stressor a really big deal, try expanding your perspective and ask yourself 'What's the long-term impact of this setback?' The answer will help to give you a sense of the stressor's significance. Take this one step further by expanding your perspective of the world at large and consider some of the other challenges that people are facing right now, such as racial violence, starvation or terminal disease.

AFFIRMATIONS

Affirmations are short, positive statements that help to keep our minds aligned with our desired path. They can serve as an anchor for the mind that tends to wander into unhelpful or negative territory when given the freedom to idle, especially at bedtime.

Guidelines for Creating Effective Affirmations

Purge the old: begin by acknowledging that your negative self-talk must be eliminated. We need to let go of the old ways first, in order to welcome the new.

Make it personal: you cannot change anyone else's beliefs, attitudes or habits but your own! Write it in your own language, it must feel comfortable to say.

Present moment statements: use present tense language. Instead of wishful statements such as "I will be so excited…" say "I am so excited that…". We are inviting our dream into reality NOW!

Be precise: avoid generalized statements, such as, "I would love to have a job one day." and say instead "I love my new position as____ at ____." Being specific is key.

Make it positive: instead of reciting what you don't want, emphasize your desire, for example, instead of "I will NOT…" try "Today I commit to…"

Include emotion: describing strong emotional states will attract your intentions to you much quicker. Use highly charged emotional words, such as adjectives like: fantastic, exhilarating, outstanding, stunning, thrilling or exciting. And adverbs such as passionately, lovingly or joyfully.

Create statements that jazz you up: Your new thoughts need to offer a sense of hope, and excitement and motivate you to take action.

Stay open to possibilities: don't be so married to your dream that you miss amazing opportunities along the way. Remain open to your future unfolding in the best possible way, which may be bigger and brighter than the current dream you hold for yourself.

Update your affirmations: keep refining your intentions as you achieve your goals!

Over time through persistent practice with affirmations, you will transform your existing limitations into a new reality of courage, confidence and freedom!

Sample Affirmations

These are generalized statements that you can tailor to your desires

I feel amazing as I grow stronger and more confident in who I am every day!

Today, I look in the mirror and choose to completely love and accept myself, just as I am.

I am happily enjoying my new loving and supportive relationship/friendships.

I relax knowing that the world is filled with goodness.

I easily and effortlessly attract abundance into my life.

I am everything that I choose to be. I am as unlimited as the endless Universe.

I let go and trust the process.

For more information on intention setting, visit www.IntentionCoins.com.

Repetition of an Affirmation (Japa)

Japa is an ancient mindfulness practice that involves a short English affirmation or a Sanskrit mantra (special word or phrase). While in traditional settings, a student would be assigned a mantra from his/her teacher based on the student's specific gifts, we can choose our own mantra or affirmation. Some examples are: Om (oneness), peace (or shanti), I am peace, I am love, I am safe etc.

Japa is done with a mala, a string of 108 beads which the practitioner, sliding fingers along each bead to keep track of their recitation. You can

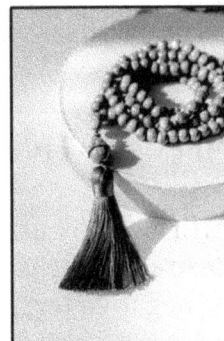

either recite your affirmation 108 times to go through the full string, or if time allows, turn and go back for a total of 216 times. This practice is wonderful for kinaesthetic learners who absorb teachings best by experiencing them through the senses. When you're done your round of japa, lay the beads down and sit for a few final moments in silence, resting your awareness on your breath.

Note: this practice complements the work done in the cognitive therapy component of this program.

PRACTICES FOR REGULATING THE BREATH AND EMOTIONS

These breathing practices can be done either sitting in an upright, relaxed position or lying back. They can be used as a precursor to mindfulness practice or as the focal point of a practice. The recommended duration for these exercises is five to twenty minutes.

One the easiest ways to harness our attention in any moment is to simply turn our awareness to our breathing. Most people have adapted to our culture of high stress, rapid speed and stimulation overload by unconsciously altering their breath. In an attempt to control our out of control lives, many people hold their breath, breathe shallowly or breathe rapidly. As you can imagine, these types of breathing create great imbalances in the body. When we breathe shallowly, like we do when we're afraid or in pain, we deprive the body of essential oxygen and energy, leading to fatigue, mental fog and anxiety. Breathing rapidly can cause hyperventilation, which happens when we start breathing very fast and release excessive carbon dioxide from exhaling more than we inhale. This can lead to feelings of light-headedness and tingling in the fingers, causing anxiety, confusion and panic.

BREATHING SPACE

Simply taking a few moments for a little Breathing Space can help to regulate the breath and calm the nervous system. We'll focus on three components of the breath: depth, pace and texture.

Let's find a comfortable seated posture and establish a restful gaze with eyes slightly open, but downcast. Bring your awareness to how you're breathing, without trying to change anything. Simply become 100% aware of your breath, moving in and out naturally, of its own accord. Focus intently on the cooling sensations of your breath entering your nostrils and the warming sensations of the breath leaving the nasal passage.

Shift your awareness now to the **depth** of your breathing, noticing how deeply the breath flows into your lungs and how fully it flows out. Encourage deep and full breathing for a few more cycles.

On your next breath, turn your focus to the **pace** of the breathing, noticing how quickly or slowly your breath travels. Does the inbreath and the outbreath move at the same pace, or does one move faster or slower than the other? Guide your breath into a steady, even pace.

On your next breath, observe the **texture** of your breath. Is your breath sharp and irregular like a rockface or smooth and soft like a meandering river? Invite your body to breathe in a slow, smooth and steady way. Don't get too caught up in doing it right. Just maintain an open awareness of this natural process known as the breath cycle. Enjoy a few more moments of Breathing Space and when you feel ready, lift your gaze and return to your life.

FULL YOGIC BREATHING

Also known as Balloon Breathing for younger children.

A full deep breath involves three-part inbreath, breathing into the belly (the lowest aspect of the lungs), the ribcage (the middle aspect of the lungs) and the collarbone region (the upper tips of the lungs). This is followed with a full and complete outflowing breath, like pouring water out of a jug. Try it a few times, breathing through the nostrils, let the breath fill the belly, the ribs and the collarbones like blowing up a balloon and then exhale, letting the breath effortlessly flow all the way out.

Note: teens can lie down and place a textbook on their belly and chest to highlight this movement of the abdomen and chest, while younger children can use teddy bears or other toys.

FALL-OUT BREATHING

Step 1: some styles of mindfulness use the exhalation as a central focus, which encourages the belly to soften and the mind to surrender. This is one of the most basic breathing habits that we often do instinctively to release stress and return to a state of (green zone) balance. Start by taking a full inhalation in through the nostrils, followed by a complete exhalation through an open mouth. You can choose to exhale either with a breathy sigh or with a vocal sigh, sounding out hhhhhaaaa, starting high pitched and dropping low. Fall out breathing, also known as waterfall breathing, helps to awaken a parasympathetic response, allowing us to 'rest and digest' as well as bring some humour into the moment with its funny sounds. Even three consecutive fall out breaths can break the momentum of negative thought pattern and set us on course for a more mindful mindset.

Step 2: 1:2 ratio breathing could easily be added here where the length of the outbreath is double that of the inbreath. Most commonly the inhalation is done to a count of four and the exhalation is done to a count of eight.

CIRCULAR BREATHING

Each breath brings you more and more present to the feeling tone within your body in this moment. Starting at the bottom of a circle, as you take deep and full inhalations, imagine your breath traveling up one side of a circle to the topmost point. As you release the exhalation, imagine the breath traveling down along the other side of the sphere to land at the bottommost point where you began. Continue breathing in a circular formation, smoothing out any pauses or breaks along the way. Attempt to equalize the measure of both the inbreath and the outbreath, beginning with a count of four in, and four out. Gradually, increase the count of each inbreath and outbreath to eight, and then with practice lengthen them to twelve.

As you continue to mindfully breathe, at the top of the inhalation you can invite a gentle pause before the breath turns over and flows into the exhalation. At the end of the exhalation, allow for a brief pause before filling the lungs with oxygen again. Let your body guide this process, as you may be awakening a dormant hunger to slow down. Pausing briefly in the spaces between breathing movements allows us to experience a beautiful inner stillness This breathing practice requires us to be attentive, patient and willing to explore new patterns, as this may feel very different from your usual breathing style.

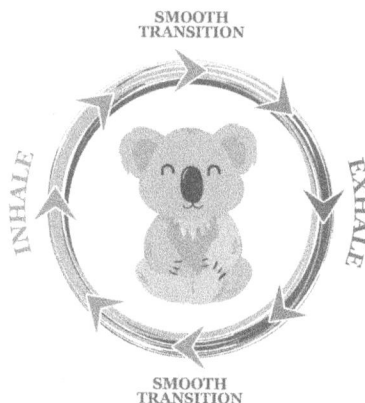

Finally, let's take this one step further to explore our lungs capacity. On your next inhale, take 18-20 counts to slide up the side of the circle and fill the lungs to their fullest capacity, expanding the space between your ribs. Pause briefly at the top of the inbreath and taking another 18-20 counts start your exhalation, slowly sliding down the other side of the circle. Keep exhaling beyond your normal range, feeling the abdomen contract toward the spine. Pause momentarily before taking in another smooth, deep breath, no rush as you pause and then exhale, another full outbreath, encouraging all the breath out of the lungs like clearing out an old stuffy basement. One more time, inhaling energy, oxygen and all things good for 20 counts. Exhale thoroughly to a count of 20, emptying the lungs of any residual toxins and stagnant breath.

Now, gently allow your breathing to return to a natural smooth rhythm with no pauses, and if you notice your new normal pattern of breathing is a little bit deeper, this is good. Most people take between 15-18 breaths per minute, and with a mindful breathing practice we can lower that rate to 7-9 breaths.

HEALING SOUNDS

Speaking calmly and using soothing words helps to calm frazzled nerves and ease emotional turmoil. The next time you feel yourself becoming emotionally triggered or provoked, try gently repeating phrases like "I'm relaxing now" or "Everything's just fine." Exhaling with Fall-out breaths to sounds like shhhh and haaa generate comforting reactions in the body. Start with a higher pitch and slowly lower your tone as you breathe out to add to the de-escalation effect.

PURSED LIPS BREATHING

The Fall-out breathing technique can be altered slightly by (inhaling through the nostrils) and exhaling through pursed lips, which helps to lengthen the outbreath and release nervous energy. With younger children, this can be likened to inhaling the smell of a flower, or their favorite scent, and exhaling the same way they would to blow out birthday candles or ignite kindling.

PRACTICES FOR REGULATING THE BODY

FIVE SECOND BODY SCAN

Within this manual are various body scan practices, which can be done by scanning with your mind's eye from head to toes, or toes to head. While the practices shared here are designed to take fifteen or twenty minutes, it is also effective to do a five second body scan anytime throughout the day, as you're doing different activities. Scan by scan, it is possible to alter your baseline of tension and recreate a new normal for how you feel inside your body. Simply turn your attention to your body and notice your scalp, face, jaw, throat, neck, chest, belly and pelvic floor. The mere practice of placing your attention on your body will help to soften hardened areas and re-establish natural full breathing.

SQUEEZE AND RELAX

Inhale, squeeze your hands into tight fists, scrunch up your shoulders and tighten your facial muscles. Exhale and relax your upper body, letting your shoulders drop and your arms dangle. Notice how your grip has relaxed and let that spread through your body. By squeezing the neck and jaw muscles past their usual tension, followed by relaxation, we help to reset the resting tone of these often-tense muscles.

HEART/BELLY CONNECTION

Adding onto the heart connection pose, with your right hand on your heart, simply place your left hand onto your lower abdomen, just beneath your navel center. This is a powerful gesture, or mudra that reminds us to honour the wisdom of our hearts, as well as the primal guidance of the gut. Placing hands on the belly also has a calming effect on the enteric nervous system, or gastrointestinal tract.

ROOTS

Sitting or standing with feet on the floor (ideally in socks or bare feet), take a deep breath in and on your exhalation, drop your awareness down into your feet. Become totally present to your feet in contact with the floor, and the floor connected to the earth. Become aware of sensations in your feet and the grounding nature of gravity, like roots of a tree reaching deeply into the soil.

This attention practice shifts awareness from obsessive ruminating habits of mind, into the lower reaches of the body. When we feel ourselves escalating into the yellow or red zone, this is a great tool for breaking momentum and bringing us back into our breathing body.

This earthly connection could be augmented by a Qi Gong practice whereby you find a seated position, slide one foot on top of the other thigh and slap the sole of the foot 30 times. Switch sides to complete the practice. This practice helps to awaken pressure points along the arches of the feet, giving an infusion of energy into your whole system.

SOOTHE YOUR SENSES

Take a ten-minute break to curl up in a cozy blanket, play soft music, soak in the elements of nature, drink a warm cup of calming tea, etc. What do your senses appreciate when you need a break from the demands of life? This ties into the trauma-sensitive practice of anchoring one's attention on an external focus through the senses, such listening to a sound, or visually focusing on an object to ground our attention in the moment when our internal world becomes overwhelming.

HEAD MASSAGE

Most body work in the western world focuses on every part of the body, but the head, the one body part that often needs it the most. Worry, fear, anger and stress all create tension patterns in the head, jaw and neck so spending time each day with a brief self-massage is an excellent way to reset the tone.

Start by removing any hair pieces and begin sliding fingers through hair from front to back, starting at the top, moving to the sides with each stroke.

Use second knuckles of your fingers to rub around the temple and side of head, where tension builds from clenching.

Rub each ear lobe, tugging at the bottom in a backward direction, then rub the head just behind the earlobes.

Just above the inner creases of the eyes, press into the brows and hold for 10 seconds, then rub from the beginning of each brow out to the temple.

Using the second knuckles again, massage the joint of the jaw in circular motions.

With one or both hands, rub the base of the skull and down the neck to release common tension.

Take a few quiet moments to be still and let the effects of this brief self-massage settle in. Close your eyes and let them sink into your skull, soften your tongue and take 3 fall out breaths. Smile, open your eyes and return to your day with renewed energy and freedom.

MINDFULNESS QUOTES

The use of short powerful quotes is a superb way of provoking thought and reflection. The following quotes can be used in endless ways. Some suggestions are

- Present one quote each week on the wall or board so its visible each day
- Quotes could be individualized and placed in a large container for children to draw from when they need guidance or reassurance.
- Quotes could be used to prompt a writing assignment that expands on its message, through a fictional story or personal reflection in their mindfulness journal. What does this quote mean for you individually? How might this quote influence our society and the world at large?
- Take the quotes (or words from each quote) and write them on pieces of paper where they can be made into prayer flags to decorate the classroom.
- This could be followed by a group discussion at the end of the week on how they incorporated the teachings of the quote into their lives.
- The author of the quote could also be researched to learn more about their life experience.

The following are a list of suggested quotes, thoughtfully following the flow of the school year, however, students might be inclined to research their own after a few months.

Week	Quote for the Week
SEPTEMBER	
1	"Deep Breaths, less stress." ~ Author unknown
2	"Gratitude pulls us out of our chosen brand of suffering so that we can see the beauty and goodness surrounding us." ~ Jenny Kierstead
3	"You can't stop the waves, but you can learn to surf." ~ Jon Kabat-Zinn
4	"There are two ways of spreading light: to be a candle or a mirror that reflects it." ~ Edith Wharton
OCTOBER	
1	"In a world that's obsessed with doing and producing, its essential that we take time each day to day dream and just be." ~ Blair Abbass
2	"Sometimes I just look up and say Thank You!" ~ Ally Donaldson
3	"If you find yourself in a hole, the first thing you do is stop digging." ~ Anonymous
4	"In the end, just three things matter: how well we have lived. How well we have loved. How well we have learned to let go." ~ Jack Kornfield
NOVEMBER	
1	"Surrender to what is. Let go of what was. Have faith in what will be."~ Sonia Ricotti
2	"The answers you seek never come when the mind is busy, they come when the mind is still." ~ Leon Brown
3	"Don't believe everything you think. Thoughts are just that—thoughts." ~ Allan Lokos
4	"Everything you've ever wanted is on the other side of fear."~ Unknown
DECEMBER	
1	"Remember to invest in RBC—Relax, Breathe and Choose!" ~ Mindfulness in Schools Manual
2	"When you first begin mindfulness, the movement of thoughts may feel like a rushing waterfall. But as you continue to apply the technique of recognizing thoughts and returning your focus to the breath, the torrent slows down to a river, then to a meandering stream, which eventually flows into a deep, calm ocean." ~ Sakyong Mipham

Week	Quote for the Week
3	"It is not death that people should fear. They should fear never beginning to live." ~ Marcus Aurelius
4	"Our brain is continuously being shaped - we can take more responsibility for our own brain by cultivating positive influences." ~ Richard J. Davidson
JANUARY	
1	"The future belongs to those who believe in the beauty of their dreams." ~ Eleanor Roosevelt
2	"Feelings come and go like clouds in a windy sky. Conscious breathing is my anchor." ~ Thich Nhat Hanh
3	"The tragedy of life is not death, but what we let die inside of us while we live." ~ Norman Cousins
4	"Every day in every way, I'm getting better and better." ~ Emile Coue
FEBRUARY	
1	"Life is about using the whole box of crayons." ~ RuPaul
2	"A mind filled with fear can be penetrated by the quality of loving-kindness. But a mind filled with loving-kindness cannot be overcome by fear." ~ Sharon Salzberg
3	"Life isn't about finding yourself Life is about creating yourself." ~ George Bernard Shaw
4	"Success is the sum of small efforts repeated day-in and day-out." ~ Robert Collier
MARCH	
1	"Believe in. yourself and all that you are. Know that there is something inside you that is greater than any obstacle." ~ Christian D Larson
2	I AM – two of the most powerful words. For what you put after them shapes your reality. ~ Unknown
3	"The creation of a thousand forests is in one acorn.
4	"Don't waste a good mistake. Learn from it." ~ Robert Kiyosaki
APRIL	
1	"In my daily commitment to self-love, I choose to love myself more than I did yesterday and to love myself even more tomorrow." ~ Mindfulness in Schools Manual
2	"Mindfulness is the noble act of making friends with yourself. Breath by breath, moment by moment, you learn who you really are." ~ Susan Piver
3	"Mindfulness is paying attention on purpose non-judgmentally in the present moment as if your life depended on it." ~ Jon Kabat-Zinn
4	"We are encouraged to bring the mindfulness we develop sitting to all of the activities that make up our lives." ~ Larry Rosenberg
MAY	
1	"Your calm mind is the ultimate weapon against your challenges. So relax." ~ Bryant McGill
2	"Beauty is not in the face; beauty is a light in the heart." ~ Kahlil Gibran
3	"Radical Acceptance is the willingness to experience ourselves and our lives as they are." ~ Tara Brach
4	"If we are peaceful, if we are happy, we can smile and everyone in our family and our entire society will benefit from our peace." ~ Thich Nhat Hanh
JUNE	
1	"Today, fill up your cup of life with sunshine and laughter." ~ Dodinsky
2	"The place to be happy is here. The time to be happy is now." ~ Robert G. Ingersoll
3	"Don't cry because it is over, smile because it happened." ~ Dr. Seuss
4	"The best things in life are not things." ~ Ginny Moore

QUICK TIPS FOR A MINDFUL LIFE

Suggestions for use:
- These can be presented as artistic statements around the classroom,
- They can be put into word art
- Students can select one and apply it to their personal practice each week
- Students can choose three tips that encompass their lifelong aspirations and live by them

1. Slow down
2. Breathe deeply
3. Witness your thoughts
4. Talk less
5. Laugh and smile more
6. Unplug more than you're plugged in
7. Watch less news
8. Immerse yourself in nature
9. Listen to silence
10. Let it go
11. Don't take it personally
12. Welcome goodness
13. Conserve your energy
14. Question your beliefs
15. Open your heart
16. Be a human BEING
17. Seek out beauty
18. Practice RBC (RELAX, BREATHE, CHOOSE)
19. Mute your inner-critic
20. Love yourself first

MINDFUL GAMES

These are great team building activities to do at the beginning of the year. They encourage students to be supportive of one another, they relieve self-consciousness by drawing their attention to a neutral external focus, they create team work, trust and a playful learning environment.

Any of these activities could be used to help learn anatomy or Sanskrit terminology if done as part of Yoga Grade 11.

Note: use larger balls (i.e beach balls) with younger grades or students with delayed motor skills.

HOOLA HOOP

Give each student a hoola hoop, spend a few minutes spinning them around various body parts to heighten their interoception. When it's time to sit for practice, they can rest it on the floor and sit inside of it. The hoop is an effective tool for clarifying students' personal space, for themselves and other students. This can represent their safe place within which they can relax, feel at ease and practice mindful awareness. Note that a yoga mat can serve the same purpose, as can a chair.

JUGGLING

Juggling is a wonderful way of harnessing the mind while developing hand-eye coordination (not to mention screen-free time). In order to do this activity successfully, the mind and body must cooperate and work together. Start with one or two light sheer fabric squares and invite students to explore with tossing them in the air from one hand to the other without letting them drop. When they're ready, they can add another piece into the mix. For the hand with two squares, one square is tucked between the ring and pinky fingers while the other is pinched between the thumb and index finger, which is tossed up first to start things rolling. After one hand tosses a square into the air, the other tosses one up so there's a square in the air at all times. Progress to crumpled balls of paper, (students could write Relax, Breathe and Choose on each one before crumpling), then progress to tennis balls.

MINDFUL WORDS GAME

In small groups of five or six, give a blank sheet of paper to each student to write down a word related to mindfulness practice, such as peace, breathing, Now, etc. Invite them to ball it up and then put it down in front of them. Start with one student throwing their ball of paper across the circle to another student, who throws it to another etc., ensuring everyone is included. Gradually add every students paper ball and when the teacher says stop, they open their paper to read what word they received.

NAME GAME

In small groups of five or six, start with one tennis ball per group. As students' toss the ball across the circle, they say "Here Erica (the name of the receiver)" and as they receive the ball, they say "Thanks Jim, here Erica." And continue for a few rounds to familiarize the group with each other's names.

MINDFUL MANTRAS

In the same small groups, instead of saying names, as they catch the ball, they say HERE, as they roll the ball they say NOW. Add up to four balls to harness their concentration. To build on this, as students catch the ball, they recite the first part of an affirmation like "I am..." and then when they throw it they recite "enough" (For example) Students can choose their own affirmation or teacher can assign it.

BREATHING ACTIVITY

In small groups, practice a breathing exercise by breathing in when you catch a ball, breath out as you throw. Keep it slow.

MINDFUL AFFIRMATIONS

The thrower says to the catcher "You are amazing" and the receiver echoes that with "I am amazing" and then passes to the next, continuing the affirmation.

This could be turned into a gratitude exercise by sharing something they're grateful for each time they catch a ball. There are many variations to this small group activity, like incorporating French language into the activity. With so much non-verbal communication, you could eventually try to do these activities in complete silence.

TOILET PAPER CONNECTOR

In small groups, one student starts with a roll of toilet paper, holds onto the end and throws it across the circle. Each student holds onto the paper before throwing it so eventually, they create a web within their group. This is a wonderful exercise for demonstrating that everyone is connected, even if we may not have much in common with them, we are all part of the greater human family.

MINDFUL MANDALA GROUP SHARING

As a class, form one circle and sit on cushions or on heels and use an item from the class as a 'talking stick'. As someone wishes to share, the stick is passed to that person, where they share a reflection or insight about the practice while others listen without interrupting and then it's passed to the next person. Not everyone needs to share but it's encouraged that over time, all will participate. Close with the chant of Om or silence.

QUESTIONS FOR REFLECTION

- There could be open discussion on how they treated themselves throughout the activities. What did they do when they dropped the ball? Were they kind to themselves or did they judge themselves harshly? This is an opportunity to observe their proficiency at mistake resilience--can learn from their goof-ups which moves them closer to success next time or will they harshly reprimand themselves, corroding their confidence?
- What about stress, was it easier when there was one ball versus five balls at the same time? Can you see how it's the same in our lives? the more things we have to juggle at once, the more stressful it is.
- Were you concerned about your grades, or relationships or your future during this game? Your troubles didn't suddenly disappear, your attention simply shifted.
- Did you notice that it became easier and easier the more you did this game? This is called practice and training our minds to be more present and open to growth and gratitude takes practice, but the more you do it, the easier it becomes.
- What other lessons did you glean from this exercise?

Six-Week Mindfulness Program

These lesson plans are designed in segments so teachers can select which components are appropriate, given the grade and maturity of students.

It is recommended that students buy a journal that they can bring with them to each mindfulness class for note-taking and self-reflection.

It is also advised to give students the following questionnaire before and after your mindfulness program, to give them (and you) a sense of their progress.

PRE AND POST MINDFULNESS QUESTIONNAIRE

Please complete this questionnaire before you begin your mindfulness practice. After completing the program, re-evaluate your responses and see if there has been any change. Rate on a scale of 1-5 where:

1	2	3	4	5
No, not at all		Somewhat		Yes, very much/often

	Score Before	Score After
Beginner's mind – I am open to learning new life skills and to making changes that allow for greater personal success.		
Exteroceptive awareness – I am aware of external stimuli, such as sensations, sights, sounds, and smells from my environment.		
Interoceptive awareness – I am aware of my inner experience, which includes what's is going on in my body and in my mind.		
Self-regulation – I am aware of my actions and the possible results of my behavior (as opposed to behaving absent-mindedly).		
Emotional regulation – I am able to identify my emotions as they arise and regulate them when I become triggered.		
Non-judgment – I am able to remain neutral about my current experience of the moment (versus being judgmental and critical).		
Non-reactivity – I allow my thoughts and feelings to come and go, without my attention getting fixated on them.		
Non-striving – I am content with my life and I am able to rest in the moment with enjoyment.		
Body/Self-Love – I have respect for the body I've been given, and I love and accept myself just as I am.		
TOTAL SCORE		

We discover the good life by taking time to slow down,
appreciate the moment, listen to our dreams, share a laugh,
and give thanks for all we have!

CLASS 1: INTRODUCTION TO MINDFULNESS

(Class length: 1hr 15 minutes)

Affirmation

Breathing in, I'm aware of breathing in. Breathing out, I'm aware of breathing out.

Supplies

- Stereo and music
- Chairs: set up in a circle with the facilitator included
- Boxes of tissues interspersed throughout the circle
- Participants can bring: a cushion, a blanket, journal and pen.
- Participants can leave: time pressures, stress, life concerns.

Welcome and Housekeeping Items (about 5 minutes)

This course is designed to be an introduction to mindfulness with the hopes of assisting you in developing your own regular practice upon course completion. Each class builds on the next so we highly encourage you to attend each week consecutively.

Teacher's Note: take the time to note where bathrooms are located and provide any other housekeeping items they might need to feel safe and comfortable.

Mindfulness Class Agreement

Use as a guide for establishing a safe and respectful class climate
- Be here: we agree to be punctual and as mentally present as possible.
- Confidentiality: we agree as a class to keep what is shared in this space confidential, (noting that all adults have a legal responsibility to report child abuse).
- One voice at a time: we agree to respect the person who's speaking by letting one person speak at a time.
- Share the mike: we agree to be aware of our tendency to speak too much or too little and to create a space where everyone can share their experiences.
- Honor our growing edge: understanding that safety is partly an inside job, we agree to honor our growing edge by listening to our physical and emotional needs and making choices that help us to feel safe.
- Respect for others—understanding that personal safety is also contingent on the class climate, we agree to practice non-judgement, non-violent behavior and tolerance.
- Seek permission first: we agree to respect other students' personal space by asking permission before we step on their mat or make physical contact. We also agree to ask permission before we offer advice.
- Group generated—brainstorm for any additions they would like to make to this agreement in order for all student to have a positive mindfulness experience.

Teacher's Note: It is advised to briefly refer back to the agreement at the onset of each class so that students are clear on what is considered acceptable conduct within a mindfulness class.

About this Program

While mindfulness practice is often done in silence, we will be interspersing our quiet time with guided visualizations with music that use our imaginations to help guide the mind into a relaxed and focused state.

Open Centering (about 5-6 minutes)

Find a comfortable seat, in a chair or on your cushion. Take a few moments to 'feather your nest' by arranging blankets and pillows. Give yourself permission to shift around until you settle into a place of ease.

Sitting tall, close your eyes and drop your awareness into your body and notice how you're holding yourself here. Take a deep breath in and consciously begin to release any held tension from your day on the exhalation. Do this a few more times, feeling your body soften and let go with each fall out breath.

Now become aware of your reason for being here…what drew you to attend this program in mindfulness?

30 second pause…

What is it you would like to achieve from this experience?

30 second pause…

Now turn your answer into an intention, for example, "I intend to learn tools for managing stress in my life."

30 second pause…

Let's allow that intention to rest in your heart space and notice how that feels. Fuel it with a few more deep, full breaths and then let it go, releasing your intention into the vast field of potential that surrounds us. Just let it all go…breath by breath, let everything go….

30 seconds of silence…

Slowly begin to return your attention to the room and your fellow participants.

When you feel ready, you can open your eyes.

Let's greet our classmates with Namaste, honouring the light within them and their intentions for being here.

Tadaa, you just practiced mindfulness!

Introductions (about 10 minutes): briefly share your name and what you hope to attain from this experience.

Teacher's Note: if the class is large, have them share in partners.

Let's start by discussing what mindfulness is not, as there are many myth's and negative ideas about mindfulness that can prevent us from experiencing its benefits.

Myths about Mindfulness (about 5 minutes)

Myth: The ultimate goal is to empty the mind and tune out.

Truth: Very few practitioners reach this evolved state of mental stillness. It is our goal rather to focus our concentration, instead of letting the mind wander and daydream.

Myth: Only special people, who are steeped in wisdom or discipline can practice.

Truth: The beauty of this work is that anybody is eligible to receive the benefits that mindfulness brings—anybody!

Myth: Mindfulness and the practice of being present is risky business, opening our minds to the possibility of being overtaken by evil spirits.

Truth: rest assured that spirits will not overtake you through this practice. In fact, you have a much greater chance of disturbing your mind with dark influences by watching TV than you do practicing mindfulness.

Myth: mindfulness is a religious cult that will try to brainwash you.

Truth: mindfulness is NOT a religion, although people around the world including Christians and Tai Chi Masters alike use mindfulness practices to deepen their studies. Mindfulness is not designed to shape or manipulate your beliefs, but rather intended to expand your consciousness by informing you of greater and greater realms of awareness. Mindfulness inspires us to be less self-serving and more humble, forgiving and compassionate toward the greater human family. In fact, by developing our awareness we become more compassionate toward all living beings, including ourselves.

Myth: Group additions: what have you heard or believed about mindfulness?

What is Mindfulness (about 5 minutes)?

The core components of a mindfulness practice include:
- Paying attention to the present moment
- Self-awareness
- Non-judgment-compassion
- Non-striving-acceptance
- Loving-kindness

Throughout this program we will explore these concepts and apply them first hand into our lives.

The Art of Paying Attention

Mindfulness, according to the great yogic master Patanjali, is 'a steady continuous flow of attention directed toward the same point or region.' It is a process of pulling away from the many external stimuli to enter a state where we are able to pay full attention to the moment. It is within this state of passive attention, where we access self-awareness. It is a state of high creativity, and interconnectedness, also referred to as non-duality, where subject and object merge into one. It is a state where we no longer experience the rain, or the wind as something separate, but rather we experience the rain and the wind, as part of us.

Ultimately, mindfulness involves the tricky practice of uninterrupted concentration that leads to a highly focused mind. Training the mind to focus on one aspect of reality, be it energy, the breath, a word or affirmation, can provide not only a sense of inner peace, but a radical transformation of our whole lives, transporting us into new ways of being and interacting with our world.

Benefits of Mindfulness (about 10 minutes)

> A wise teacher once said, "There is nothing more threatening to our well-being than the unguarded mind."

One day, Prince Siddhartha Gautama, who later became the Buddha or Awakened One, saw a holy man who had been meditating in the mountains for many years. Despite his impoverished physical state, he had a strangely serene look in his eyes. The Buddha suddenly realized his life of privilege was bereft of meaning and his search for the truth of existence and for inner peace had begun. After many years of wandering the land, on a severely restricted diet, Siddhartha came to the realization that neither a life of excess or of renunciation was the path to peace, but that a lifestyle of moderation was the way. This began his teachings on the middle path. We are all, more than ever, searching for the same peace of mind that the Buddha longed for. However, this inner state of peace and serenity is largely unattainable in our materialistic, hectic world.

There's good reason for this curiosity toward such peace of mind that seems unattainable. The reality is that the average person is bombarded with 20,000 – 70,000 thoughts each day, that's one thought every five seconds! Added to this equation is the fact that most of these thoughts are unproductive, distressing, driven by craving, anxiety and obsessive thinking AND they're repetitive.

The more we unintentionally give our thoughts free reign so that our thoughts and the emotions associated with them are controlling the way we conduct our lives, the more we become locked in negative feeling patterns such as guilt, shame, resentment, anger, anxiety, fear etc. No wonder we're a culture riddled with stress, anxiety, and depression—we're letting our minds run the show! As a result, many of us feel out of control of our lives, with little to no peace or inner rest.

With mindfulness practice, we start questioning the validity of every thought, which allows us to disrupt our usual (and often harmful) thought patterns. We begin to work with the 'monkey mind' that leaps from branch to branch or thought to thought. This practice can be likened to spring cleaning, where we take inventory of our thoughts and sift through the junk. Mindfulness brings our unconscious thoughts into conscious awareness, where we can gain greater control of our thoughts, emotions and reactions.

Gradually, over time, we enter the state of neutral, non-judgmental, compassionate awareness, and have a direct experience of the moment. This experience of being truly present is a homecoming to our natural state, or ultimate reality. We all have the potential to wake up, to see life clearly and experience peace of mind; we just need to start where we are right now.

As we become more skilled in the practice of mindfulness, we gain a greater ability to harness the power of our minds. Imagine yourself in the forest at dawn, attempting to find your way home. Would you want to have a weak, dim flashlight in your pack or a powerful, focused laser beam of light? Mindfulness sharpens our mind to become the laser beam.

Mindfulness practice gives us the gift of aha moments, when our current, limited view of reality expands and we suddenly understand life in a vastly different way. A busy mind creates confusion and frustration, whereas a calm mind brings clarity and solutions.

Mindfulness brings our unconscious beliefs to the surface for our conscious mind to assess. Unpleasant feelings, thoughts, traumas and emotional states rarely go away on their own. By sweeping them under the rug, they just gather dust and continue to limit our experiences. Instead of letting our unconscious beliefs dictate our lives, through mindfulness practices we are able to heal the issues we've kept hidden and move on to enjoy the many rich aspects of life. We become skilled at thinking the thoughts we want to think, when we want to think them.

Through mindfulness training, we learn to control our emotional reactivity, empowering us to respond more rationally to stressful situations that would otherwise send us into a panicked frenzy.

When we are distracted and living out of the moment by worrying about our next appointment or clinging to a past experience, we are not present to the gifts within the present moment. Becoming more mindful enables us to enjoy each moment more, so our food becomes more flavourful, flowers become more fragrant, sunsets become more beautiful, and the touch of a loved one's hand becomes that much more tender. In other words, our experience of life becomes richer, sweeter and fuller.

Through mindfulness, we learn to be more tolerant and compassionate with ourselves. We become aware of our shared humanity, that everyone experiences birth and death and the time in between is often filled with imperfect, even messy life lessons. As we grow in our ability to be more compassionate to human suffering, we become more accepting of ourselves and others. This leads to a genuine desire to help relieve suffering in the world and we become more interested in positively contributing to life.

Mindfulness can even save us money! The lingering joy of being fully present eventually far surpasses the temporary and superficial joy of the material world.

From a research perspective, mindfulness in school-based contexts reveals the following list of core benefits

- Improved concentration and focus
- Greater emotional regulation
- Decreased stress, anxiety and depression
- Enhanced impulse control and self-awareness
- Increased resilience
- Improved ability to respond skillfully to challenges
- Increased empathy, compassion and understanding of others

We'll be touching on these benefits in the following weeks of mindfulness lessons.

How to Practice Mindfulness

In a nutshell, the practice of mindfulness is the practice of restful awareness, where we learn to become aware of ourselves with each passing moment. It is also known as metacognition, the ability to think about thinking, or become aware of one's awareness. This includes, awareness of one's posture, breath, and sensations as well as one's thoughts, conditioned perspectives and emotional reactions to life situations. With greater awareness comes a greater ability to assess one's behaviour after the fact and learn from each life experience. This has been referred to as dual awareness where we learn to be immersed in the experience, while maintaining an observer's perspective and watching the moment unfold. Simply put, mindfulness helps us to be more aware of our thoughts and our actions moment by moment.

With that, we can practice mindfulness within a controlled, still environment as well as in the midst of the busy-ness of life's activities. When starting out, it is best to find a quiet, clean place that is void of distractions such as technology and socialization.

The body is conditioned to nap when we lie down so whenever possible find an upright position. Sitting in a chair, or on the floor with hips properly supported and hands resting on the thighs, we begin by closing our eyes, or gazing slightly downward.

Using mental focus, we relax each body part, beginning at the top of the head, scanning down to the feet.

We then turn our attention to our breathing, regulating the flow of the in breath and the outbreath, letting the diaphragm relax and move freely As air travels in and out of the lungs, we learn to smooth out the breath, equalize the inhalation and exhalation and deepen each breath we take.

Drawing our awareness away from the lure of the outside world and its constant distractions, we turn our attention inward.

When distractions arise in the mind and we are tempted to disconnect from the present moment experience, we can use any number of tools to draw us back, such as breath awareness or an affirmation. Training the mind to return to its focus of choice takes dedication but over time, like strengthening a muscle in the body, this capacity will become stronger and stronger. The mind will gradually become identified with the object of your choosing instead of wandering from one random thought to another, which doesn't serve your highest good.

The Practice of Being Non-judgmental

"Mindfulness is an impartial watchfulness, it does not take sides."
Ven. Henepola Gunaratana, *Mindfulness in Plain English*

We often hear about mindful practices making people more peaceful and calm. While the results of a mindful practice may lead to that, mindfulness itself is neutral and non-judgmental. This practice teaches us to keenly pay attention to the traffic in our mind as it arises, without judging it. Mindfulness is not necessarily wise, kind, loving, or happy, but it has proven to generate those qualities as a result of the practice. The more conscious we are of our thoughts, the more aware we become of just how judgmental we are. We might even catch ourselves judging how judgmental we are!

This judging nature is a deeply seated survival instinct that helped us to quickly categorize things within our field of vision as dangerous or benign. But this judgmental pattern has its pitfalls, causing us to become biased about certain people and situations which narrows our perspective. When the judgmental lens is turned on ourselves, it can damage our self-worth, lead to obsessive, perfectionistic tendencies and create a whole lot of pain. Therefore, in efforts tame the minds inclination to judge and criticize, we'll be approaching the practice of mindfulness with a **non-judgmental, self-accepting and patient** mindset. Over time, as you introduce a few judgment-free moments here and there, you'll notice that judgment and criticism don't actually propel you forward, but rather hold you back from living your best life. With a bit of practice, you'll be surprised by how good you feel, how much richer your relationships are and how much more progress you can make by assuming a self-accepting, compassionate approach to life.

Mindfulness Roadblocks

While the framework of mindfulness is fairly straight forward, it's common to experience sharp turns, speed bumps and roadblocks on the path to present moment awareness. It's important to be aware of these factors so you can be prepared for them, not surprised or discouraged by them when they do arise.

The following are just a few roadblocks and experiences you may encounter on the path to mindfulness

- You may resist the inward journey and have difficulty being present to your body and your breath
- You may have body memories arise (energy patterns that have become trapped within your cellular make up)
- You may have thoughts; rapid, recurring thoughts
- You may experience boredom, frustration or agitation
- You may succeed at repeating your word of choice (known as mantra) or an affirmation such as 'I am peace'
- You may have thoughts and affirmations occur simultaneously
- You may slip into a mindful state of spacious, peaceful awareness
- You might even fall asleep

When to Practice

Morning and evening correlate with our body's quieter rhythms. Because our bodies and minds long for stillness, we just need to provide the time and space for it. Like any exercise program, routine is key, as we are training the mind and it responds to practice much the same as muscle does, gaining strength and endurance.

Length of Practice Time

The effects are cumulative, so even 10 minutes here and there help to train the mind. As you begin to notice benefits you may rise a bit earlier to sneak in 30 minutes, and eventually you'll feel ready for an hour of practice, either all at once or 30 minutes in the morning and 30 minutes in the evening or late afternoon.

Mindful Moment (about 5 minutes)

Close your eyes and give yourself time to absorb this information: 20,000 – 70,000 thoughts a day, many of which are repetitive. Consider the idea of training your mind, just like we do our bodies. Let's take just 30 seconds to watch the rambling of our thoughts, as though watching a movie without clinging to the story line. Since the breath is intimately linked to the flow of consciousness, focus on breathing smoothly and notice what you notice.

- Silence for 30 seconds...
- Slowly open your eyes and return to the room.

This practice is a simple bare bones awareness of the moment and our breathing. Recite quietly to yourself: "Breathing in, I'm aware of breathing in. Breathing out, I'm aware of brea thing out."

That 30 seconds is a snapshot of our present state of mind. When beginning anything new, it is essential to accept where we are, as there is no other place to start.

Confucius said, "The journey of a 1000 miles begins with a single step." And we have officially begun the journey of awakening through mindfulness.

Quiet Reflection (about 5 minutes)

In your journal, write down your intention for being here.

Now take the next five minutes or so to record all the reasons why you can't or haven't practiced mindfulness before.

Title your page with: *The reasons I can't practice mindfulness are...*

Partner Sharing (about 5-7 minutes)

In pairs, take a few minutes to mutually share your responses and highlight your two most compelling reasons. Together, brainstorm solutions or ways around these reasons for not practicing mindfulness.

Thank your partner and come back to your nest.

Mindful Practice (7-10 minutes)

Settle into your comfortable seat again, sitting tall but not rigid. Relax the muscles of the neck and face, the back, the entire body. You can keep your eyes slightly open, gazing downward or close them.

Begin by noticing your breath and follow its rhythm in and out of your body.

Inhale and visualize your inner landscape expanding, exhale and allow your muscular network to relax deeply. As we move through the various aspects of our being, maintain a smooth and steady breathing pattern.

Silence for 1 minute...

Become aware of your external environment, the people sharing this space, the distant sounds of vehicles, wildlife (human or animal☺), fans or heaters.

Now become aware of your internal space, noticing sensations in your body, including those that are pleasant and those that may be causing you discomfort or even pain. Just notice, without a need to fix or change your present situation in any way.

Turn your attention to your thoughts, and observe the constant stream, the coming and going of thoughts and judgments, without losing yourself in them.

Now observe any feelings that might be present here...pushing nothing away...just accepting your feeling state, as it is in this moment.

See if you can get a sense of the core of your being here, the essence of who you really are. This is sometimes referred to as your true nature or your essential self.

Through the practice of present moment awareness, we gradually enter a state of oneness, where we feel connected to the wholeness of life. Take a moment to feel this connectedness to all beings, all creatures and all things.

When we expand our awareness in this way, we feel free and spacious, because awareness is endless, quiet, still and vast enough to hold the chaos of life without being altered or affected by it. Continue to return to being present to this spacious, infinite state of awareness that has no boundaries, no limits.

Breathing smoothly and deeply, explore the fullness of your breath, filling the belly, the ribs and the chest with the inbreath, then emptying the lungs completing with the outbreath.

With each in breath, affirm to yourself that you are 'breathing in' and 'breathing out.' Breathing in, breathing out, breathing in, breathing out.

Silence for 5 minutes...

Gently draw your attention back to your body and your breathing. Take a moment to rest here. Slowly open your eyes, joining the group again.

Group Sharing About the Practice Experience

Closing

Your Omwork for the week is to do 30 second full yogic breath practices, where you follow the inbreath to completion, then the outbreath, three times a day. If you are inclined to go longer, do so.

Reflection Questions

During mindfulness practice, when you are watching your thoughts like viewing a movie on a screen, ask yourself who is doing the watching?

What happens to the depth, pace and texture of the breath when you pay attention to it?

Write in your journal each evening, reflecting on new insights and challenges or recording questions.

CLASS 2: THE WISDOM MIND

(addressing the mindfulness component of self-awareness)

Affirmation

> With humility and respect,
> I honour my highest teacher,
> The wisdom within me.

Welcome and Announcements

Centering Mindfulness (about 7-10 minutes)

Find a comfortable seat, in a chair or on your cushion. Take a few moments to 'feather your nest' by arranging blankets and pillows to create optimal comfort. Give yourself permission to shift around until you can settle into a place of ease.

Sitting tall, close your eyes and drop your full awareness into your body and notice how you're holding yourself here. On the exhalation, consciously begin to release any held tension from your day. Do this a few more times, feeling your body soften and let go with each fall out breath.

30 second pause...

Let your breath find its natural rhythm now and just observe its ebb and flow for a few moments...what sensations do you notice as the breath enters and exits the body? Are you a bit more familiar with your breath this week?

Silence for 1 minute

What do you notice about the pace and rhythm of your breathing when you turn your attention to it? Try to keep your inquiry focused on your body, there's no need to get too intellectual.

30 second pause...

Now take a moment to reflect on who's doing the observing here? What part of you is actually following the breath and consciously staying present to the moment? Can you give this part of yourself a name or a title?

30 second pause...

Returning to your breath again, let your exhalation just fall out of your mouth, let it all go...breath by breath, let everything go....

30 seconds of silence.

Slowly begin to return your attention to the room and your fellow participants.

When you feel ready, you can open your eyes and greet your classmates, honouring their intentions for being here.

Brief check in (about 10 minutes)

How was your first week of mindfulness practice?

Are you able to see how mindfulness can improve your health in the many ways outlined in class 1?

Discuss Class 1's Reflection Questions (15 min)

What happens to the rhythm and quality of the breath when you pay attention to it?

The Observer Effect

According to Quantum Physics, the process of observing a system changes the system, and therefore makes the observer part of the system being observed. So, in terms of our breathing, the moment we pay attention to it, we change it, typically by slowing it down. This simple process of observing the breath is a profound tool for enhancing our wellbeing.

Follow up on the reflection question from Class 1

During mindfulness practice, when you are watching your thoughts like viewing a movie on a screen, who is doing the watching?

Teacher's Note: Invite student's answers.

The Witness

Teacher's Note: In cases of mental illness or trauma, therapy may be necessary before going inward in this fashion. Additionally, our inner voice of wisdom is ALWAYS loving and kind, so if a student notices violent messages being communicated, it is recommended s/he seek support from a professional.

Let's explore the observer effect further. By simply becoming aware of a situation, the situation changes instantly. This reflects the power we hold within our own minds to change our reality. In this course, we'll call this the witness.

By becoming aware of our inner witness, we become capable of curbing emotional upheaval, understanding negative behaviour, changing thought patterns and rewiring the mind. We see proof of this by simply drawing our attention to our breathing and observing its pace and depth change instantly. The witness is the part of us that remains steadfast, stable and calm, unaffected by life's challenges.

But the alternative is true as well, since our minds also host an inner roommate who busily fills our life with thoughts, and most of the time, negative, worst-case scenario thoughts. This part of our mind doesn't stop thinking, not even for a second!

In fact, the average person is said to have between 20,000-70,000 thoughts per day, that's about 40 thoughts per minute! This constant mental chatter can lead to great distortions in our perceptions and cause deep distress in our lives. The witness, however, is able to watch the mind drum up reasons to be anxious, fearful, or resentful, and not be pulled in to the many story lines. This ability to observe our thoughts then, gives us the power to choose to identify with the wise and peaceful voice.

Renowned teacher Ram Dass shares a profound conversation he had with a heroin addict After picking up the phone, he was greeted by a hysterical, suicidal voice on the other end, begging Ram Dass for help. He instinctively appealed to the part of this woman who dialed his number, asking to speak with her wisdom mind, or the one who bears witness. Once he made contact with that part of her, Ram Dass was able to help her navigate the crisis.

The witness allows us to see life without the usual conditions and biases that tend to sway or color our reality. The witness, which enables us to watch the drama of the mind unfold, is like a portal to our inner voice of knowing. This inner voice, which is a source of boundless wisdom and strength, can lead us toward healing and peace, so long as we learn to trust its guidance. In order to make contact with this inner voice of wisdom, we must first quiet our thinking mind to listen more deeply.

Expanded awareness

One day a teacher wrote a V on the board and asked the class what it was. They all replied confidently, "It's a bird!" After applauding their quick response, the teacher said, "No it is not a bird, it is the sky with a bird flying in it." This story is a great metaphor for the practice of mindfulness, as often our focus becomes so limited that all we see is the object of our attention, like a challenge or problem that we can't seem to overcome. Through mindfulness, we learn to expand our perspective to see the sky, which represents the pure unbounded quality of awareness.

10 Minute Mindful Practice

Let's take a few moments of silence to practice accessing the witness by observing the busyness of your mind. Over time you'll notice that your mind is able to slow down, shifting from the rapid-fire 40 thoughts a minute to an open spacious awareness of the moment. Just like training a muscle in your body, training your mind takes practice, so this may not happen right away. Stay as present as you can in a curious, non-judgmental way and just see what happens.

Three minute pause...

There is so much good occurring all around us each and every day, but our untrained mind keeps us mired in dread and drama. As we learn to step out of the daily drama and watch the goings on in our minds, we realize that our thoughts are not always an accurate reflection of reality. With this realization comes great freedom. Once we understand that the thoughts we think do not define our reality, nor do they define who we are, we can then open our hearts to truly experience the miraculous, the beautiful and the humorous side of life.

Take another few moments to sit quietly, breathing smoothly, simply watching your thoughts float in and out of your awareness like clouds in the sky. It is not our goal to empty the mind and NOT think at all, but to observe our monkey mind, that swings from branch to branch, from thought to thought, distracting us from the moment and all its richness.

Three minutes of silence...

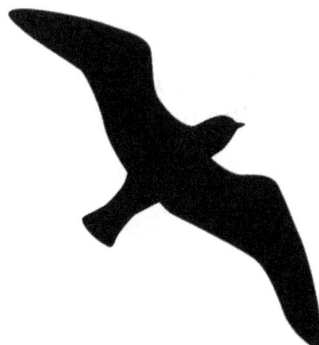

From this new perspective of the witness, you can then break the cycle of destructive thought patterns by creating space in your consciousness for peace to settle in.

Returning to the room, let your body shift around or move in the way you need to.

Teacher's Note: As a class, discuss their experience and any reflections they have on the concept of dual awareness and the witness perspective.

Mindfulness practice on the inner voice (5 min)

Reflect on a time in your life when you were able to hear your inner voice of wisdom. What message was it communicating? Did you listen and pay attention? When our inner voice communicates, it will always bring a special quality to the moment, and these moments are often remembered for our entire lives.

In a culture that has become overly focused on the intellect, on rational thinking and logic, we have lost our connection to our deep sense of knowing. Our inner voice also becomes clouded by fear and self-doubt, and mindfulness enables us to see these blocks so that we can release them.

Can you gain a sense of where this knowing occurs within you? Is it in your third eye, your heart, or maybe even a gut feeling?

Give yourself this time to quiet your thinking mind, imagining the intellectual part of your brain, the cortex, quieting down and resting at the base of your skull. Now become aware of your breath and practice fall out breathing, where we inhale through the nose and exhale with a long sigh. Two more times, inhale deeply and exhale let it go, inhale and exhale with a haaa…inviting yourself to land right here, in the present moment.

Through your awareness, let yourself connect to the place inside where all your answers reside. No need to search for anything. No need to force anything. Simply soften your outer being and sink into the truth within you. The following is an affirmation for acknowledging this very important part of our existence:

With humility and respect,
I honour my highest teacher,
The wisdom within me.

Journal (5 min)

Choose one area of your life that you're finding particularly challenging. What would your highest teacher, the wisdom within you advise? How might your engagement with your inner voice enhance your life?

Group Discussion (10 min)

In groups of three, share with each other your relationship with your inner voice of wisdom. Where does it reside in you—the head? The heart? The gut?

With humility and respect,
I honour my highest teacher,
The wisdom within me.

Closing Quote

At any time in our lives, we can assume the perspective the witness, which remains clear of daily drama and abides in present moment awareness.

CLASS 3: MAKING PEACE WITH THE MOMENT

(addressing the mindfulness component of non-striving)

Welcome and Announcements

Centering breaths (7-10 min)

Find a comfortable seat, in a chair or on your cushion. Take a few moments to 'feather your nest' by arranging blankets and pillows to support your positioning. Let yourself shift around until you can settle into a place of ease.

Sitting tall, close your eyes and drop your awareness deeply into your body and notice how you're holding yourself here. On the exhalation, consciously begin to release any held tension from your day. Do this a few more times, feeling your body soften and let go with each fall out breath.

30 second pause...

Let your breath find its natural rhythm, just simply enjoy its ebb and flow...As we did in class 1, you can accompany the in-breath with the silent affirmation "Breathing in" and as you breathe out, silently affirm "Breathing out."

Silent pause...

Can you make contact with the part of you who witnesses the breath, moment by moment? Let's take a moment to quiet the intellectual, thinking mind and access the radiant wisdom of the heart.

Silent pause...

Take a moment here to reflect on your week and notice how these principles have percolated into your life...

Let's take three deep breaths together and on our third exhalation we'll join in the sounding of Om, the sound of universal oneness.

AAAUUUUMMMmmmmmm...silence

Brief check in (about 10 min)

How have these teachings affected your life, for example, the way you face adversity, conflict, or your inner dialogue?

Theme for Today

Making Peace with the moment, instead of making the moment peaceful.

Most of us grow up in our western culture receiving few or no truly effective strategies for coping with the challenges and uncertainties of today's world. The most common way we attempt to deal with life is by seeking to control it, believing that if we can only fix this or that 'problem', it will go away and we'll finally be able to rest in peace and comfort. But that peace and comfort never arrives because life is constantly presenting us with new challenges, which is the nature of being human. And so we spend our lives, striving for control of the uncontrollable. When we realize we can't control life, we view ourselves as failures and seek to escape life through sensory pleasures such as food, drink, entertainment, technology or work etc.

When we accept the natural conditions of life, the unchanging principles, we can begin the process of *making peace with the moment* instead of trying to make the moment peaceful.

1   Everything changes and ends. Everything in life has a cycle of arising, sustaining and falling away. Everything.

2   Things don't always go according to plan—we don't actually have the control we like to think we have.

3   Life is not always fair or comfortable—we all have different life situations and challenges, so fairness is an unreasonable expectation. Ps; if you're too comfortable you're likely not growing.

4   People are not always loving, honest or loyal—yes, that includes you too. ☺

Quiet Moment (5 min)

Take a moment to reflect on the above conditions and notice where they are at play in your life right now Take a few minutes to write down concrete examples of each of these unchanging principles in your own life, for example, a time when you've fudged the truth, or someone betrayed you.

Share with a partner a time when you've experienced any or all of these in your life.

As a class, share a few responses as to how acceptance of life's conditions actually changes your experience of life? Did anyone feel more at peace, relaxed? Perhaps somewhat depressed? Did anyone feel disappointed by life? Many of us have been misinformed about the nature of life, especially if our well-intentioned parents protected us from the simple truth that nothing is permanent and that everything changes. We are often thrown surprises, since people (even those we know and love) are inconsistent.

Mindfulness practice (about 25 min)

Let's begin our mindfulness practice with **Guidelines on physical posture during sitting mindful practice** When our physical body is resting in true alignment, we are more likely to settle into a state of mental and emotional harmony. These are general guidelines to follow to the best of your ability, while keeping in mind that many people access relaxed brain states in a variety of different body forms. You do not have to be able to turn yourself into a pretzel in order to experience mindful awareness!

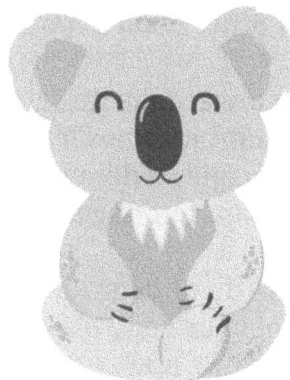

Spinal Alignment

Choose a position that feels suitable for you right now. Unless you are living with an illness, we advise that you sit up, with your spine tall, since the body is conditioned to equate lying down with sleeping. Initially, you may find it very difficult to sit up straight unsupported by a backrest so feel free to sit back and rest your spine against the chair. We do however want to gradually strengthen the muscles along the spine so that we can sit at the edge of a chair or on a cushion without support. The position of sitting tall gives feedback to the part of the brain stem involved with wakefulness, sending the message to stay alert.

Take a moment now to find an upright position, gently leaning from one sit bone to the other, visualizing your energy anchoring into the earth. Recite quietly to yourself as you shift side to side: "Here Now...Here Now...Here Now."

Legs and Feet

If sitting on a chair, the legs can either be bent at a 90-degree angle with feet on the floor, and if the feet don't rest completely on the floor prop them with blocks or books. Sitting in a crossed legged fashion, with your seat elevated is another option. This traditional posture with the legs crossed symbolizes our commitment to sitting for a period of time. With our legs crossed, we can't move about. If your legs are crossed and your knees are higher than your hips, elevate the hips with extra support, allowing the hip flexors to release and the knees to drop. You might also feel more comfortable with support beneath the knees as well.

Note that very few westerners can sit safely in Full Lotus, Padmasana, so we advise that you keep the soles of your feet perpendicular to the floor, instead of upward facing.

Take a moment to relax the hips and legs, letting your lower body surrender to gravity.

Arms and Hands

Slide your upper arms back so they hang in line with the torso. This will be the most restful position for the neck and shoulders. With your hands resting on your thighs, you can choose to have your hands open faced to the sky or turned down toward the earth. Try both and see which option feels energetically aligned with your state of being. If you have a favourite mudra, or hand position, you can assume that or simply let your fingers relax in a slightly curled position.

Take a moment here to let your arms hang gently with your hands resting peacefully in your lap.

Head Position

Ideally the head is positioned directly over the spinal column so the crown of your head aligns with your pelvis, or more specifically, the perineum. This prevents compression in the neck. It may require some effort to uphold this posture since many people today commonly have a slumped spine with the head thrust forward. Unconsciously and over time, we develop this posture from driving, working at the office, bent over our electronic devices, or straining to see the screen.

Take a moment to tuck the chin in toward the throat, as you lift the base of the skull away from the neck. Now let the chin rise until it comes level to the floor and visualize your ears aligned over your shoulders. Finally, imagine a divine hand tugging at a string attached to the top of your head and gently lift your head, creating a quality of lightness throughout the neck and spine.

Notice how you feel here, from the tip of your toes to the top of your head. Can you feel the physical and energetic harmony of your body placed in a sacred way?

Shift your awareness to your breathing now, exhaling with a sigh a few times to relieve any discomfort or unnecessary tension. Ideally, this is a position you can comfortably sustain for a few minutes.

Now imagine yourself as a container rather than a physical body. Imagine this container to be large enough to hold all of life's challenges, disappointments, and struggles. Do so from your heart center with compassion and ease When we're immersed in chaos, we can expand our awareness and hold space for life's challenges with calm acceptance.

As we let go of the illusion that it's possible to create a perfect, pain-free life, we stop the constant striving to make the moment peaceful and learn to make peace with the moment, as it is. Sense the peace that comes with this perspective.

Take a few moments now to rest in silence, enjoying the harmony of your physical body and the expanded nature of your energetic being. Notice how it feels when you drop the belief that you need to change anything about your life.

Who you are right now is enough. You are enough. Allow your life, with all its imperfections to be enough, as it is. There's nothing to change or fix. Let yourself make peace with the moment. As we sit for the next few minutes, you can silently recite the mantra: I am peace. 'I am' is recited on the inhalation, 'Peace' on the exhalation.

Silent pause...

Slowly return your attention to your natural breathing pattern and to sensations in your body. Take a moment to relax here before we transition out of our mindfulness practice. When you feel ready you can open your eyes, stretch out your legs and fold forward, letting the head gently release toward the earth.

Closing

Group Discussion (about 10 min)

Q and A on the mindfulness process and physical posture.

Closing Quote

I make peace with the moment, and accept my life, as it is. Peace, Peace, Peace.

CLASS 4: EQUANIMITY

(addressing the mindfulness component of non-striving)

Welcome and Announcements

Centering Meditation (about 7 min)

Find a comfortable seat, in a chair or on your cushion. Take a few moments to 'feather your nest' by arranging blankets and pillows to support your positioning. Let yourself shift around until you can settle into a place of effortlessness.

Let's review the **postural guidelines for sitting mindfully**. Go ahead and close your eyes or lower your gaze and drop your awareness into your body. Notice how you're holding yourself here, are there muscles that are unnecessarily engaged that you could relax? Become aware of the alignment of your spine and notice the natural curves of the spine. Sit tall, imagining someone tugging on a string attached to the top of your head, while at the same time, feel yourself root down into the earth through your sit bones. Your legs can be bent in a simple seated position in a chair or crossed legged. Let your upper arms hang along-side your torso, with relaxed hands and fingers resting in your lap or on your thighs. Finally, slightly tuck your chin and draw your head back so the crown finds its alignment over the pelvis.

Fall out breaths

Take a few deep, fall out breaths, inhaling through the nostrils, exhaling with a sigh. As you exhale, feel any unnecessary tension evaporating into space. Do this a few more times, feeling your body soften and let go with each fall out breath.

Circle breathing

Now close your mouth and let's explore circular breathing, where we breathe in, traveling up along one side of a circle and out through the nostrils, flowing down the other side of the circle. Slow and smooth inbreaths, followed by an even slower and smoother outbreath, your breath creating a circle with each full cycle.

Now at the top of the inbreath, pause and hold for a moment, and then let the outbreath cascade out like a waterfall. Inhale again through the nose, for a count of four and hold your breath for a count of four, and exhale for a count of four. Inhale up one side of the circle for 1, 2, 3, 4, hold at the top for 1, 2, 3, 4, exhale for 1, 2, 3, 4 and add a pause here for 1, 2, 3, 4. Continue to this breath pattern for a few more cycles, imagining your breath tracing the shape of a circle.

Silent pause...

Return to your natural breath now, and in this state of open awareness, reflect back on life's givens or conditions that we discussed last week:

1. Everything changes. So long as it's alive, everything is growing, changing and will one day die.
2. Things don't always go according to plan. Spontaneity is always sprinkling spice into our lives.
3. Life is not always fair or comfortable, we all have our own unique lessons to learn.
4. People are not always loving, honest or loyal. We must approach our relationships with compassion and model integrity.

Take a quiet moment here to reflect on your week, observing how these higher truths have influenced your life...

Silent pause...

Let's take three deep breaths together and on our third exhalation we'll join in the sounding of Om.

Group Discussion (about 10 min)

Invite sharing about their week and any progress, insights or challenges that arose. Did you reflect on life's unchanging principles? Do they make sense to you?

Theme: The Practice of Equanimity and Observing Craving (about 15 min)

Today's class builds on last week's theme of making peace with the moment by exploring the challenging practice of equanimity. Equanimity, a Latin word that means "even mind", speaks to the art of maintaining a balanced mind that lies at the root of mindfulness practice. The practice of equanimity enables us to stay neutral (in the green zone) in the presence of an emotional trigger or a craving, which stands in stark opposition to our brain's ancient wiring to react and take action. Detaching from the pull of the craving mind also works against our western culture, which profits from our addictions to entertainment, on-line shopping, gaming, social media, internet surfing etc.

The ego is part of our mind that is active when we experience fear, jealousy, competition and craving. Ancient sages called this the unquenchable thirst or the ever-hungry belly, as we can spend our whole lives jumping from one thing to the next in attempts to satisfy the ego. But like a bucket with a hole at the bottom, the ego is never satiated, never satisfied. This is demonstrated daily in our culture obsessed with consumerism and material gain, even at the cost of our financial stability and the balance of the environment.

Through the practice of equanimity, we become aware of a state much deeper and enduring than the petty requests of the ego. When we tap into this state of stillness, we realize that our need for status, to be the best, buy that expensive car, or have the perfect body, are not true needs at all. While money and material gain may bring more enjoyment, they don't always satisfy our longing for lasting happiness. One just has to look at the many unhappy celebrities whose personal lives often spiral out of control into drug addiction and other destructive behavior. As we become more aware of the richness that exists within the simplicity of the present moment, we begin to realize that our enjoyment of life is not contingent on material things. After all, studies show that we don't wear 80% of the clothes in our closets!

By simply observing and bringing an awareness to our desire to want more, or different, we liberate our inner resources that have been busy feeding the ever-hungry belly of our craving instinct.

Here's the key point to remember, craving and peace generally don't co-exist. When we're in a state of wanting something, we're removed from the present moment and from our peaceful nature. When we are consumed by craving, we are often overcome with feelings of discontent, frustration and anger. Less is truly more when it comes to finding peace.

Dopamine is an important neurotransmitter in the brain that drives us toward reward and pleasure. It's helpful to be aware that the teenage brain tends to have a lower dopamine baseline than the adult brain, so teenage behavior can seem dramatic and extreme because the brain needs more stimuli to get the same pleasure reaction. This is yet another reason for developing equanimity and training the mind to stay present in all moments, even the neutral, peaceful one's, when it's not scanning for threats or reaching for pleasure. With equanimity, we're able to abide in a deep ocean of peace, instead of being thrown around at the surface by the tumultuous storms of pleasure and pain, likes and dislikes.

Note: craving is not to be confused with our heart's desire, which is an essential inner drive that often calls us to fulfill our life's purpose.

Quiet Moment (about 5-7 min)

Take a moment to conjure up a time in your recent memory when you were consumed by craving. Let yourself become completely absorbed in this state of wanting and needing. What is your feeling state here? Record your findings.

Mindful Practice (about 15-20 min)

Let's begin our practice by settling into a position that can be sustained for a period of time. Guide your breath to slow down and let the in-breath flow deeply into the base of the lungs, then feel it filling the rib cage up to the collarbone region. Exhale and relax the temple of your body while keeping the spine erect and the head nicely balanced and level.

Encourage your body to relax and your mind to rest here in the present moment. Allow your life situation with all its details to just be as it is.

As you sit, you may notice preferences arise, craving your phone or attention from so and so. Notice the energy it consumes within you and how it preoccupies your mind. Equanimity breaks the cycle of suffering by creating separation between you and your craving mind. In the open state of awareness, we can be present to our cravings, without reacting impulsively to them. We can do this by practicing the acronym RBC, relax, breathe and choose. Let's start by bringing to mind, something that we tend to crave on a day to day basis, like a certain food, your phone, an energy drink, Netflix, etc. As you think of this craving, give the intensity of your craving a score, with 1 being the lowest and 10 being the most intense. Notice how your body feels in the presence of craving; tight, tense, maybe even stressed at the need to satisfy it?

Give the craving space to exist, without trying to push it away, let's introduce RBC by relaxing your body, letting any tension dissolve, like ice melting into water. Notice what number the craving is now...Now let's breathe deeply and mindfully for a count of ten; inhale and exhale for 1, inhale and exhale 2, inhale and exhale 3, inhale and exhale 4, inhale and exhale 5, inhale and exhale 6, inhale and exhale 7, inhale and exhale 8, inhale and exhale 9, inhale and exhale 10. If your mind wandered, that's okay, the more you practice following your breath with your awareness, the better you'll become at it. After our simple breathing practice, notice your craving now, what score would you give it? Let's keep breathing mindfully as we tune into the vast openness of awareness. Observe your thoughts and sensations coming and going, without chasing after pleasure or pushing away the unpleasant, just let them flow like leaves floating downstream.

After some time, you may notice a sense of serenity, peace and contentment arise, as you rest in equanimity, an even, neutral state of mind...Notice what score you would give your craving now? Completing the final letter in the acronym RBC, which focuses on choice, how might you choose to act after giving your craving space and infusing it with awareness?

With practice, you'll gradually feel greater and greater degrees of freedom from the enslavement of your cravings Gently deepen your breathing now and rest here for a moment before opening your eyes, returning to the room.

Small Group Discussion (about 10 min)

In your groups, share your experience with the practice of replacing craving with the RBC acronym of relax, breathe and choose. Did you learn anything about your wanting nature?

Closing

Your true self is the part of you that exists beyond the constant craving to want more. Your true self is unlimited, bright and peaceful.

Om-Work

Continue to carve out quiet time for mindfulness and contemplation.

Observe the craving instinct of the ego and record your insights.

Remind yourself of equanimity by choosing a peaceful photo as your screen saver on your phone.

CLASS 5: LOVING KINDNESS

Centering Practice

Teacher's Note: give each student a battery-operated candle and ask them to turn it on.

Welcome everyone, let's gather around and find a comfortable seat. Align your body in a way that supports an attitude of wakefulness and attention, but also allows for a softening to occur within. Take a few deep breaths and let yourself settle into your mindfulness posture (reviewing the posture guidelines if necessary). With fall out breaths, imagine each exhalation releasing held tension in your skin, your muscles, your organs and other deep tissues. Sigh it all away, a few more times.

Silent pause...
Let's explore the spaciousness that exists between our ongoing streams of thought, and just linger there in that awareness.

We tend to spend so much of our lives seeking change, wanting to make our lives better or different. We are taught to believe that the next moment holds something more for us and so we keep striving for that illusive something that exists in the future.

Mindfulness gives us time each day to step out of that striving frame of mind and allows our lives to just be as they are.

Silent pause...
Just let it all be...let this moment be enough.

3 minute silent pause...
Like the flame of a candle remaining undisturbed by the wind, we are cultivating the ability to calmly abide in the moment, through the many storms, full of emotional upheaval, disappointments, cravings etc.

By sharpening our moment-to-moment awareness, we drop the need to reach for the next moment and start to embody our physical selves again. When we soften physical tension, which naturally happens when we rest in the now, we allow our life force to course through us and a love force to fill the heart. We learn that to truly feel and experience life in our bodies is what it means to become fully alive.

Many of us attempt to protect ourselves from the pain of human suffering by emotionally shutting down and turning away from others in need. But authentic love, which we all long for, can only be felt when we open to the suffering of others and feel their pain. This is the nature of empathy. We are not separate from others, we are more the same than we are different and attempting to isolate ourselves only causes pain and loneliness. One person's suffering is all of our suffering and waking up to this truth will help us to heal on a collective scale.

Today we are exploring the practice of Loving Kindness.

We tend to categorize people into three groups

1. Close friends, family and those we care about, usually accompanied by a feeling of attachment
2. Those we don't like, usually marked by a sense of aversion or repulsion
3. People we don't know, usually accompanied by an attitude of indifference

The key is to develop equanimity, a beautiful word that means balance and composure, which we practiced last week. When we experience equanimity, our biased preferences fade and we can approach all people with the same degree of genuine compassion. In the end, we recognize that everyone suffers and all anybody really wants is to be happy (some people go about it more skillfully than others). Compassion, which naturally arises from loving kindness, is born from a wish to release others from their own misery.

Let's recall the first and fourth essential truths

- Everything changes and
- No one is ever loyal and loving all the time.

While we may feel affinity toward one person now, everything is impermanent. The people we know and love today may one day become our enemy. The people we deem our enemy today, may, one day, turn into friends. Such is the nature of life. Through the practice of equanimity, we are able to see the futility in both repulsion and attraction.

Enemies as Our Best Teachers

Story of the Tibetan Tea Boy

One day a great master was asked to visit a neighboring community. He gathered his personal belongings and got ready for his trip. His students eagerly lined up with the hopes of being chosen to accompany him on his journey. When the same boy was chosen again, the students began to grumble and complain. Upon returning, one student courageously approached the leader and asked: "Dear teacher, why do you continue to choose the same student to travel with you?" The leader replied: "I choose that boy because he disturbs my peace of mind, therefore his presence gives me the opportunity to practice inner balance and loving kindness toward all beings."

Although we don't need to be close friends with those who rub us the wrong way, we can practice observing our reaction to them with neutrality and kindness. By learning to be present with and process disturbing emotions such as hatred or resentment, we are then able move closer to finding peace in our minds and hearts.

This loving-kindness exercise leads to a natural uprising of compassion in the heart, which leads to freedom from past grievances and love for ourselves and others.

We'll start by directing this practice at ourselves, then move to the easiest group of people to send loving kindness to and progress from there. Let's begin by offering this phrase to ourselves:

May I be happy just the way I am.
May I be healthy in body and mind.
May I be at peace with whatever comes.
May I be filled with loving-kindness.

Repeat it once more (this short form may make it easier to remember):

May I be happy.
May I be healthy.
May I be at peace.
May I be filled with loving-kindness.

Pause for two minutes...

Now visualize a friend or family member whom you care for and recite the following phrase to them:

May you be happy just the way you are.
May you be healthy in body and mind.
May you be at peace with whatever comes.
May you be filled with loving-kindness.

Again, this time using the short form:

May you be happy.
May you be healthy.
May you be at peace.
May you be filled with loving-kindness.

Pause for two minutes...

Visualize a person whom you know but have neither affinity nor aversion toward, like an acquaintance you see regularly but don't know very well. Recite the phrases to them:

May you be happy just the way you are.
May you be healthy in body and mind.
May you be at peace with whatever comes.
May you be filled with loving-kindness.

Again, this time using the short form:

May you be happy.
May you be healthy.
May you be at peace.
May you be filled with loving-kindness.

Pause for two minutes...

Visualize a person whom you feel a sense of anger or dislike for (you may want to start small and leave deep triggers for a time when you're more experienced). Remind yourself that this exercise does not exempt their behavior or make it okay, but that we do this to help free ourselves from pain. Anyone who hurts another is either unaware or in deep pain themselves and so we offer this phrase in light of wishing peace to all:

May all beings be happy just the way they are.
May all beings be healthy in body and mind.
May all beings be at peace with whatever comes.
May all beings be filled with loving-kindness.

Again...

May all beings be happy.
May all beings be healthy.
May all beings be at peace.
May all beings be filled with loving-kindness.

Pause for two minutes...

Close the loving kindness exercise with this phrase: When we are able to rouse an equal sense of compassion for all beings, we have perfected the practice of unconditional compassion.

Take five minutes to reflect in your journal about your experience with loving kindness. Spend the first part just noting your experience and then take a few minutes to record where you can see your life being enhanced by this exercise.

Suggested power-point notes:

While most ordinary people focus on personal happiness, it is through compassion for others that we develop meaningful relationships with others.

The wise teacher Shantideva once said, "All joy in this world comes from wanting others to be happy and all suffering in this world comes from wanting only oneself to be happy."

By opening our hearts to all people, we step beyond the illusory veil of separation and we radiate great love and empathy for all.

Group discussion (7-10 minutes)

In groups of three, discuss Shantideva's statement and share examples from your own life. Then discuss any counter opinions you might have about this statement (like what about caring for ourselves?).

Invite the class to exchange three hugs before leaving (always optional).

CLASS 6: THE OLD "ME" AND THE NEW "WE"

Find a comfortable seat, in a chair or on your cushion. Take a few moments to 'feather your nest' by arranging blankets and pillows to support your positioning. Let yourself shift around until you can settle into a place of ease.

Go ahead and close your eyes, dropping your awareness deeply into your body and notice how you're holding yourself here.

Our Evolving Human Community

When the ego, or the small separate self is in the driver's seat of our lives, we live from an "I, me, mine" perspective. Put a group of I's together and we have a community of I's, who are exclusively "Me" focused. Here, we live life with the motivation to get something, with a belief that there is not enough of anything. This reflects a fundamental fear of death, of our life force being extinguished. While it may appear real, it is just a belief, and a limited one, not an accurate reflection of our true nature.

As we expand our awareness, we become present to the life force energy that animates all beings. This impulse is calling us to live in a more integrated, conscious fashion and to fulfill our highest potential through the service of others. In yoga, service to others is called karma yoga.

By shifting from the old "me" to the new "we", instead of living separate lives involving you and other, we create a sense of connectedness where there is no more 'other'. There is no longer an in crowd and out crowd, no more friends and enemies, but a new "we" culture that is built on unity and harmony. We create one home on earth for all, based on inclusion.

It is said that the Universe is a holograph, a construct created in large part by the mind. Our thought processes directly influence our physical world, and our level of awareness directly determines our social networks.

Sustainable cultures place the creative principle of the Universe at the center (like the tribe in Avatar). We must continue to grow and expand our life perspectives, flow with the river, and evolve with change. As our planet becomes more and more taxed by our greed and violence, we are faced with the pressure to evolve and re-emerge as a newly awakened society. It is now time to create communities that include everyone, a culture that leaves no one out.

Group Mindfulness Practice

In groups of four or five, sit on chairs so we're all at the same level, in a close circle. Everything arises, sustains and falls away, including every breath, every thought and even our lives. We are going to practice mindfulness together and verbally share our moment-by-moment experiences. In order to do this successfully, we're all going to have to demonstrate maturity by following the instructions, cooperating with one another and respecting others physical boundaries.

Let's start by dropping into the rhythm of deep breathing. Let yourself fully arrive here in this moment with your classmates in this space. Feel free to turn your gaze downcast or close your eyes. As you become mindful here, notice if you start to fixate on the silence, which we tend to want to fill to ease any discomfort. Instead, notice this collective silence as being both empty, with no distractions, and full, with everyone sharing this experience…

Shared silence is something very powerful that few people experience together. Our work is to remain inwardly present to the flow of our breath and the sensations in the nasal passage as the breath flows into your lungs and out, while also being outwardly aware of others doing the same thing. Simply be here, with dual awareness, observing yourself, while observing the collective experience.

As thoughts arise, don't resist them, become aware that your mind has wandered and bring it back to sensations of the breath. No matter how many times it wanders, bring the mind back with kindness and patience.

The Dalai Lama once said, "There are two days of the year that nothing can be done. One is yesterday and the other is tomorrow. Today is the right day to love one another, believe in yourself, and live your life."

As a group of individuals, you are invited to ponder the deepest spiritual question people of all faiths and philosophies have asked for millennia, **who am I?**

We have been advised by our ancestors to 'Know thyself' and some have even gone so far to say that 'The unexamined life is not worth living.' In yoga, there is a saying 'You are That' which means you are part of your neighbor's life, you are part of nature, and you are the Universe! Can you feel this interconnectedness with all that exists? As thoughts and insights arise, feel free to speak them out to your group, just one or two words at a time.

Pause for two minutes...

The next big question on life is: **what do I want?** This question, if we dig deep enough beyond superficial cravings of the ego, indicates our highest core values and our deepest desires. Embedded within the layers of your heart lies your destiny, and your greatest contribution to the world in this lifetime. That said, it's natural to want the basics of life as well, such as financial abundance, healthy friendships and a loving partnership. Listen attentively to what arises for you and again, freely share a word here and there as it feels right. **What do I want?**

Pause for two minutes...

The final question, which reminds us that we are not just here to serve our own needs, but that we have a responsibility to assist others on the path of life as well, is: **how can I serve?** What is my purpose? We are all born with unique gifts that we are meant to share with the world. We could see this as our divine contract with the great creative force that made us. How are you meant to enhance the world with your unique gifts and experience? **How can I serve? What is my purpose?**

Pause for two minutes...

Now, let's become present to the dreams and visions that each one of your classmates have just declared in this moment. Imagine the answers to their questions like seeds within the soil of their being, one day sprouting and growing into full bloom. Visualize your circle as a beautiful collective flower, blossoming with the gifts you all possess within you. Imagine the clouds of confusion and uncertainty clearing above you so that the warm, glowing rays of the sun can pour down over you. Your circle is now glowing radiantly with warm, golden solar energy, helping to nurture the blossom of your dreams.

Group Sharing

Ddiscuss what arose for you from these questions.

Coming back together as a group, take a few long, slow, centering breaths, bringing your awareness back into your body. We'll close this session with an Irish poem that wishes the sun to shine upon you and guide your way home.

May the Long Time Sun (Snatam Kaur sings a beautiful version)
"May the Long Time Sun
Shine upon you
All love surrounds you
And the pure light
within you
Guide your way on..."
Debrief as a class on this group mindfulness practice. How was that experience for you? Did you feel supported by your circle? Were you distracted? What answers came to you? Do you have any further questions? If so, good, keep reflecting and paying attention because your questions and the answers to them will continue to change throughout your lifetime.

INDIVIDUAL MINDFULNESS LESSONS

The following individual lessons can be used as independent mindfulness practices throughout your day.

LESSON 1: THE BODY SCAN EXERCISE

Introduction

The body scan is a mindfulness exercise that brings the body into our awareness. Scanning the body helps us to become aware of our body's needs, which we have become accustomed to ignoring in the western world, spending far too much time in our heads. It should be clarified that this practice is not a physical practice that requires any action. Contrary to a movement practice, here the body rests in stillness and becomes the subject of our undivided, non-judgmental attention.

Tuning into the body in such a way greatly enhances interoception, our ability to perceive and understand our internal landscape, including our organs, muscles, skin, energy levels etc (see the segment on interoception for more details). For this reason, the body scan has proven to have many health benefits, like reducing blood pressure, relieving pain, releasing muscle tension, regulating the breath and soothing our nervous system.

Mentally, this practice is effective for cultivating concentration and for quieting the tendency to ruminate, which happens when we obsessively worry. Ruminating leads to a stress response, which compromises our health on many levels. Becoming aware of the various parts of your body while tethering your awareness to the breath will help to disrupt any negative thought patterns.

This is a practice of noticing what is, without attaching or attempting to change anything. If you become distracted or lose focus, simply let go and return to the process again and again.

We'll scan from your feet to your head, and all you need to do is relax into a comfortable position, either supine or sitting and enjoy. You may notice a warmth arise in areas that you're focusing on, like a surge of energy. As your mind concentrates on aspects of your body, your circulation will actually increase in that area, bringing healing where it's needed.

Body Scan Practice

Let's start by simply tuning into your breath, inviting it to flow in and out of your lungs easily and effortlessly. You may notice it slowing down, which brings feelings of relaxation and calm. Become aware of your body, especially where it makes contact with whatever is supporting it—be it your bed, the floor, a chair—just notice how it feels to be supported. Let the density of your body surrender to the grounding force of gravity.

Let's move on to exploring different parts of the body, starting with the lower belly. Draw your attention to the navel area and watch how the breath lulls this part of your body into a soften state. Watch it expand on the inbreath and deflate on the outbreath, an effortless constant motion. Follow the complete pathway of your breath, as it travels in through the nostrils, down the throat and into the lungs, with a slight pause and then follow the breath as it flows out of the body through the nostrils. A few more times, focusing your full attention on the natural, miraculous function of your breath.

Drop your attention now to your toes, notice any sensations here, feel free to wiggle them for a moment to emphasize the feeling within your toes. Notice the pads of the feet, feel the arches, the heels that bear your weight when standing and the ankle joints that connect your feet to your legs.

Notice how your calves feel, and your knee joints. Observe your thighs, the front and back of your thighs, the inner and outer thighs. Let your legs relax and melt into your support like warm butter. Ask yourself if you're holding any unnecessary tension in your lower body and allow it to let go with your next exhalation.

Sense where your legs join with your pelvis. Notice how you're holding your pelvic floor and release any unnecessary tension. Move your awareness to your lower abdomen. Feel your body just breathing itself, without any effort on your part. Become aware of the organs within your abdomen and the rhythm of your heart beating in your chest. Ask yourself, "Am I contracting the muscles in my belly or chest? Can I relax this area of my body?"

Notice the expansion of the ribs as you breathe in and the release as you breathe out. Listen for the sound of the breath, your mind following this wave-like motion. Become aware of the full length of your spine and let it soften into its support, just feeling your own body.

Notice your shoulder joints and your armpits, your upper arms, your elbow joints, your forearms, and your hands. Become present to your fingers and notice if you're holding any tension in your grip. Notice your neck and the base of your skull where your head rests on your spine. Witness your scalp, your face, your forehead, the muscles around your eyes, your jaw, your teeth and your tongue. Are you clenching the muscles in your face and scalp? Gently invite your body to relax.

Sense the skin over your whole body smoothing out, your breath flowing easily and deeply, as your body rests in stillness and peace. If it's time for sleep, let yourself drift off into a deep slumber for as long as you need to, feeling restored upon awakening.

And if it's time to continue with your day, gently return to wakeful awareness, feeling refreshed and alive from this nourishing exercise. Returning to this room, become aware of the sounds around you and wiggle your fingers and toes. If you're lying down, gently roll over and rise to sitting. Take a deep breath in, exhale as you open your eyes and smile, noticing how good it feels to be connected to your body and the present moment.

Note: if time allows, proceed through one of the mindful movement practices with the intention of maintaining this centered, grounded focus.

LESSON 2: MINDFULNESS FOR DEPRESSION

"The present moment is filled with joy and happiness. If you are attentive, you will see it."

Thich Nhat Hanh

Mindfulness can be done anytime, anywhere, and given our brains negativity bias, it's definitely a protective measure we could all benefit from implementing into our daily routine. Have you ever wondered why the one criticism stands out over the dozens of encouraging comments? Take heart, it's not just you, the human brain is wired to have a greater reaction to negative and nasty news than to positive, inspiring news (just look at Trump's popularity). Our brains evolved in this way for good reason as we once needed to fine tune our attention to danger in order to survive. And survive we have. Although our lifestyle has changed dramatically over the years, our brains have not, and therefore, still lean toward a pessimistic perspective. Rick Hanson describes this mental phenomenon as clinging to negativity like Velcro while letting positivity slide off like Teflon. The exciting and rather new field of neuroscience has revealed that with a little intention and attention, we can actually redirect this negative tendency to a more positive outlook. This ability to change the patterning of our brains is called neuroplasticity.

Negative-positive Ratio and Relationships

Not only does this inborn safety mechanism of focusing on negativity affect our own lives, studies show that our relationships require a certain amount of negative to positive interactions in order for them to last. More specifically, we need to exchange about five positive interactions for every negative each day in order to feel nourished by our relationship connections. If you find yourself struggling to maintain healthy relationships, awareness of this positivity/negativity balance may help.

For the sake of our own mental health and for the longevity of our relationships, it is essential that we learn to recognize the goodness in our everyday experiences. Researchers advise that when we experience something positive, that we pause and absorb it into the depths of our being for about 30 seconds, which is equivalent to three or four deep breaths. By consciously welcoming goodness into our lives and staying on the lookout for things that foster wellbeing, optimism and faith, we build a bank of positive memories that we can draw from anytime we need a boost. There is a yogic term sukha, that refers to ease and comfort, so let's practice "soaking in the sukha" each day of our lives (taken from Girl on Fire Empowerment).

By letting the positive experience linger in your awareness for a period of time, you're boosting happy hormones and familiarizing yourself with positive feelings which gradually alters your negativity bias. Instead of letting the weeds consume your garden of awareness, choose to focus your attention on the flower blossoms.

Student Activity 1

Take 10 minutes to walk your school property and look for pleasurable encounters (like a flower, a crisp apple, a hug from a friend). When you find it, pause for about 30 seconds, allowing your senses to fully enjoy this experience of goodness. Let it infiltrate your whole system. Take a photo of your positive experience and document how you felt after mindfully letting yourself soak in the sukha of this simple pleasure.

Student Activity 2

"The person at the top of the mountain didn't fall there."

Vince Lombardi

Draw a mountain with a snow peaked tip and write in the body of the mountain one of the difficult emotions you're facing in life. Write on the peak, the healthier solution that will help you to feel victorious. Some examples are: negativity and gratitude, self-doubt and confidence, envy and self-love, comparison and peace, hopelessness and vision etc.

Additional suggestions:

- Create an affirmation, for example: I inhale peace, and exhale comparison.
- Write a story about your life's journey from the base to the peak.
- Lead a field trip to a local mountain and climb it together, using affirmations during the hike and have students write a reflection on the experience.

Teacher's Note: if time allows, proceed through one of the mindful movement practices with the intention of maintaining this centered, grounded focus.

LESSON 3: THE PRACTICE OF GRATITUDE

People who have near death experiences or cancer diagnoses often report that their lives have changed for the better since the experience because they now realize just how precious life is and they fully capture the moment in a way they never did before. We are taught in our culture that the moment is not okay, and that we must strive to achieve and accumulate before we can enjoy it. As Shawn Achor, author of the Happiness Advantage, simply puts it "Success first, happiness second." But this approach is flawed because we don't stop to recognize when we do succeed and achieve, and so we live a life of striving, never arriving.

Mindfulness practices enable us to press pause on the constant striving and exercise santosha, or contentment, the same feeling those who have near death experiences have. This is not to be confused with laziness or living without direction. On the contrary, contentment gives us permission to live fully by embracing the moment as it is, with a grateful heart. Speaking of grateful, when you're feeling discouraged or depressed, when your life seems stagnant, or even when you're upset and angry, there is one simple secret that can turn it all around—the practice of gratitude.

The practice of gratitude as a tool for happiness has been mainstream for years. Long-term studies support gratitude's effectiveness, suggesting that a positive, appreciative attitude contributes to greater success in our work, health, sport and business.

Gratitude, or the practice of being grateful and appreciative, is one of the most powerful ways of attracting goodness into your life. Gratitude aligns your awareness with what you truly want in your life and how you wish to feel. Have you ever wondered why you spend so much time on the points of frustration in your life, instead of envisioning a solution or better situation? With our brain's negativity tilt, it's easy to become caught in the web of negativity, victimhood and constant complaining, which only lead to feelings of hopelessness. If you want to feel angry, continue to think about the things that erupt anger within you. If you want to feel depressed, focus all your attention on the depressing aspects of your life. If you want to feel victimized, harness your awareness on the stuff that's not working in your life.

Gratitude is not a blindly optimistic approach, where we ignore the dark realities of life. It's more a practice of consciously choosing to rest our attention on the good. Pain and injustice exist in this world, but when we focus on the gifts of life, we are rewarded with a greater sense of well-being and happiness.

Therefore, if you want to feel uplifted, healthy, peaceful and content, turn your focus on the factors in your life that support these states of being. If you want to generate forward momentum in a positive direction, start focusing your energy on the good things in your life, as few as they may seem in the moment.

Even in the worst of days, when it appears that everything is going wrong, there is always something to appreciate. Sometimes, it may just be the fact that you're still breathing, or that you have a big toe, or two if you're really lucky. Gratitude changes the momentum of any situation by invoking the powerful energy of appreciation. When we express appreciation and gratitude, we expand the energy of the heart. The heart is known as the strongest electromagnetic center in the body, so involving the heart in the practice of gratitude creates great shifts within and around you. Being grateful inspires generosity, which opens the doors for love to flow. If you want to free yourself and energize your life, gratitude has no equal.

While its benefits are undeniable, an attitude of gratitude can still be difficult to sustain since our minds are trained to notice what is broken, unfulfilled or lacking in our lives. For gratitude to reach its full healing potential in our lives, it needs to become more than just a word, it needs to become a habit.

That's why practicing gratitude is essential. When we practice giving thanks for all we have, instead of complaining about what we lack, we start training the mind to see life as an opportunity and a blessing. As you practice gratitude, an inner shift will occur, and you may be delighted by how content and hopeful you feel.

There are many things to be grateful for: colorful autumn leaves, legs that work, friends who listen, chocolate, fresh eggs, warm jackets, free wifi, the ability to read, roses, our breath and butterflies, to name a few.

Student Activity

Despite the challenges you may be facing right now, there is ALWAYS something to be grateful for in every moment. Let's practice soaking in the sukha (ease and comfort) by reflecting on your recent past and list off five things that you are grateful for having received or experienced:

1.

2.

3.

4.

5.

If that took a long time to fill out the short list above, you're likely succumbing to the brain's stone-age negativity preference. The remedy? You guessed it, keep practicing! Take a moment to reflect on your life right now and let your mind wander to the things in your life that you're presently grateful for:

1.

2.

3.

4.

5.

Finally, think about your future dreams and all that you hope to receive and achieve. Stay with the attitude of gratitude as you list them off here:

1.
_____
2.
_____
3.
_____
4.
_____
5.
_____

This exercise is not intended to diminish or trivialize your difficulties, but rather to show you that there is light amidst the darkness, you just need to open yourself to it. As annoying as it may sound, there is always someone out there who's worse off than you and this gratitude exercise helps to provide perspective.

As your awareness of the power of gratitude grows, you will effortlessly attract more goodness into your reality, which will shift your perspective from feeling victimized to feeling supported.

Additional Suggestions for Practicing Gratitude

- Keep a gratitude journal in which you list things for which you are thankful for as part of your morning and evening routine. You can make daily, weekly or monthly lists. Greater frequency leads to better success in creating a new habit, but just keeping the journal where it's visible will remind you to think in a grateful way.
- Make a gratitude collage by drawing or pasting pictures.
- Practice gratitude around the dinner table or make it part of your family's bedtime ritual.
- Make a game of finding the hidden blessing in a challenging situation.
- When you feel like complaining, make a gratitude list instead. You'll be amazed by how much better you feel.
- Notice how gratitude is impacting your life. Write about it, sing about it, dance about it, paint about it.

Gratitude Invocation

Gratitude is a feeling we experience in the heart.

Gratitude is inspired by acts of kindness.

Gratitude is the spark that lights the flame of love in our relationships.

Gratitude is often directed toward someone who is not physically present, but present within our hearts.

Gratitude is an eagerness to share goodness with another, free of the need to be thanked.

Gratitude is an openness to receive goodness from another, free of the pressure to give back.

Gratitude is a mindset, which attracts our dreams and nurtures our faith.

Gratitude is one of our highest states of being.

Gratitude pulls us out of our chosen brand of suffering so that we can see the richness around us.

Gratitude opens us to the awareness of a sacred presence that supports us everywhere and always.

May we fill our minds with gratitude, our hearts with gratitude, and our dreams with gratitude.

Namaste

Teacher's Note: if time allows, proceed through one of the mindful movement practices with the intention of maintaining this centered, grounded focus.

LESSON 4: STRESS AND ANXIETY

By Kelly Humphreys, School Psychologist and Mindfulness Teacher

> If your emotional abilities aren't in hand, if you don't have self-awareness, if you are not able to manage your distressing emotions, if you can't have empathy and have effective relationships, then no matter how smart you are, you are not going to get very far.
>
> Dr. Daniel Goleman

If you are in the teaching profession, it will be no surprise to hear that teaching is one of the most stressful jobs in the world. So much so that the National Commission on Teaching and America's Future reports that 46% of all new teachers in the US leave the profession within 5 years. What's more, the number of students entering school with deficits in social-emotional development and self-regulation skills has increased substantially over the last 15 years, with one in five who struggle with mental health challenges such as anxiety and depression. Sadly, only about 15% of these actually receive the help they need and the majority of this 15% who get help are accessing it in schools.

But the light shining through our darkened reality seems to arise from contemplative, self-awareness practices, such as mindfulness. In fact, research consistently shows the correlation between measures of social-emotional competence and later measures of psychological health. Therefore, from the standpoint of a school psychologist, it makes every bit of sense to complement any psychological service with an arsenal of mindfulness teachings.

When dealing with mental health, it is important to be able to identify the difference between two of the main challenges children face today: stress and anxiety. Many people confuse the two because the symptoms are very similar.

Common symptoms of both stress and anxiety:

- Rapid breathing
- Headaches
- Nausea
- Heartburn
- Lethargy
- Rapid heart rate
- Muscle tension
- Sweating
- Chest Pain

Let's take a closer at each both stress and anxiety to help identify the differences between the two.

Stress is known as a response to daily pressures from the external world. With stress, a person knows what the stressor is (ex: project, test, exam, presentation) and it's a reaction to something happening in present-time. Everyday stress is associated with feelings of frustration and overwhelm. Stress in the right proportion can be neutral for our health, and even beneficial to our lives, inspiring change and growth. But too much stress for an unbroken period of time can turn into chronic stress and the results can be devastating. Chronic stress can lead to:

- Chronically tired, digestive upsets, headaches, and back pain
- Affects the blood cells that help you fight off infection
- Increases blood pressure and risk of heart attack
- Triggers behaviors that contribute to death and disability, such as smoking, alcoholism, drug abuse, and overeating/under-eating;
- Makes it harder to take steps to improve health, such as giving up smoking or making changes in diet.
- Increases risk of cancer

For children, the impact of chronic stress can cause the following:
- By age 4 years, stress hormones may be doubled compared to peers in emotionally stable homes
- They take longer to calm themselves
- More health problems (especially coughs/colds)
- Less responsive to new things
- Lower overall academic achievement
- Display antisocial behavior and aggression
- Difficulty regulating their emotions
- Difficulty focusing attention
- Greater risk of pediatric depression/anxiety

Chronic stress sends our sympathetic nervous system in overdrive, so we end up living in survival mode. Our pre-frontal brain shuts down and we become frustrated and angry, which leads to 'red-zone' inappropriate behaviour.

> Between stimulus and response there is a space In that space, lies the freedom and power to choose our response In our response lies our growth and freedom.
>
> Victor Frankl

Anxiety

Although stress frustrates and overwhelms and can be very harmful, it does have an upside. People in the midst of stress generally feel that if they roll up their sleeves, they can tackle the specific stressor and feel better.

Anxiety on the other hand, engenders a global sense of fear and helplessness, by fueling the belief that life is uncontrollable and not going to get any better. Anxiety is one of the adverse effects of stress; it is the process during which a person becomes worried and apprehensive of what lays ahead. When we experience anxiety, we become less aware of what we're anxious about in the moment and the reaction becomes the problem. Anxiety is a reaction to something that may happen at a future date or may never actually happen at all.

Therefore, anxiety is a disorder of the future, consumed by worry about worrying. But as you and I both know, most of what we worry about never comes to pass. Given that stress is something we can generally deal with, if we can turn anxiety into stress, we can deal with it effectively because we have more tools available. One of the most common reactions to anxiety is avoidance, like a child refusing to go to school. When a child feels anxious about going to school, the most instinctual thing to do is to avoid it, but it only gets worse the next day, quickly creating a vicious cycle.

Instead of escaping and appeasing children, we need effective tools to help them deal with anxiety and stress and failure and disappointment. What mindfulness teaches is ways in which we can handle difficulty, not avoid it. What we tell ourselves about situations set off certain reactions in our brain. It all starts with thought, which then leads to physiological reactions.

The way mindfulness helps is by teaching us to pay attention, on purpose, without judgement. It strengthens our internal skills that contribute to mental-emotional balance, like teaching us to respond instead of react. Mindfulness is considered a practice because this ability to respond doesn't just appear, it is cultivated through practice. Mindfulness makes us more aware of our thoughts. When we become aware of our thoughts, we realize that they're usually not that positive or productive.

Just like a fire fighter needs to learn how to fight fires before being placed in an emergency situation, we need to practice mindfulness techniques in advance so when we become triggered or stressed, we can access our tools. We need to learn how to manage stress that is an inevitable part of being human. Stress accompanies almost every new challenge, good or bad.

Knowing how to "de-stress" and practicing when things are calm can help children and adults get through challenging times ahead. Mindfulness and self-regulation practices, therefore, are best taught when students are in the 'green zone', feeling calm and relaxed and not triggered. Learning to take deep breaths in the midst of a stressor cannot be learned in red zone. Stress management works best when used regularly, and not just when under pressure.

Ultimately, our behaviour stems from our biology, the more we understand the brain, the better equipped we are to deal with mental- emotional issues. A toaster has more instruction than we have for our brains, but that's slowly changing today.

Note: if time allows, proceed through "Mindful Movement practice – Anxiety Calming Class" with the intention of maintaining this centered, grounded focus.

LESSON 5: MINDFULNESS AND THE BENEFITS OF UNI-TASKING

With over 18,000 studies conducted on the practice of mindfulness, it is undeniable that mindfulness can enhance our quality of life by bringing more enjoyment to our everyday moments. But is mindfulness also able to give us more of those moments by extending our lifespan? From an individual standpoint, absolutely, with its ability to reduce stress related ailments, boost our moods and give us effective tools for dealing with emotional crises, it is reasonable to conclude that mindfulness can boost not only the quality, but the length of our lives as well.

What's more, practicing mindfulness teaches us to notice when our stress levels rise and what the culprit is, which usually involves jamming the moment so full that we fragment our attention into little pieces. Life today is ridiculously demanding with literally thousands of things vying for our attention in any given moment. While many of us pride ourselves on how much we can do at once and how quickly we can do it all, the hard facts on multi-tasking are harrowing.

Research has revealed that our brains don't actually multi-task at all, they just shift focus from one area of the brain to another, depending on the demands. So what's really going on when we're doing an assignment, checking social media and preparing for work at the same time? We're not actually doing all these things at once but rather swiftly changing our focus, which we can do in a mere 1/10th of second. Now you may be saying "Big deal, you do what you gotta to do to get it all done, right?"

Well, if we look a little deeper into this, we learn that multi-tasking may actually be disastrous for our overall health. For most of us, the moment we add a diversion to our attention, it increases the demand on our nervous system. With each new demand we inflict on our system, the more stress we experience. The more stress hormones our system releases, the greater the risk of developing stress-related health conditions such as heart disease, obesity, diabetes, anxiety and depression to name a few.

At some level we are wired for stress, it makes us feel alive, and for some, stress is the antidote for boredom. But the next time you're engaged in the juggling act of multi-tasking, take notice of how you're breathing. Chances are, you're not breathing at all and unfortunately, we humans need to consume oxygen and release carbon dioxide in order to survive. In fact, this breath-holding pattern sends your system directly into fight/flight/freeze, which we mistakenly interpret as being productive. In reality, it's downright dangerous.

But take heart, there is a remedy to this insane, multi-tasking lifestyle we've maladjusted to, and the answer is pointing to the practice of uni-tasking (uni meaning one). Uni-tasking is the art of on doing one thing at a time and devoting your full attention to it. It all starts with a commitment to shifting from a stress-laden lifestyle to a more sustainable way of living.

The following are three simple steps to set you on your path

1. When you choose to take on anything that requires concentration (such as working, socializing or especially driving), make the conscious choice to be fully present. Turn your phone on 'Do not disturb', park other responsibilities, set a timer if you need it and tune into the task at hand.
2. When the urge to multi-task arises, you can write it down as a reminder for later, take a few deep breaths and return your focus to your current activity.
3. Take stock of your life and your schedule. If you're feeling maxed out and chronically stressed, you may need to refine your calendar so that it reflects your intention to live

in a more healthy, balanced way.

As you embark on your uni-tasking approach, you'll soon notice incredible benefits seeping into your life. When you're eating, you'll be truly tasting. When you're conversing, you'll be truly connecting. When you're resting, you'll be truly relaxing. It won't be long before you see yourself becoming calmer, more creative, more patient, more joyful and surprisingly more productive.

Teacher's Note: if time allows, proceed through one of the mindful movement practices with the intention of maintaining this centered, grounded focus.

LESSON 6: THE FOCUSING WALK IN NATURE

The Power of Nature

Although most people today spend over 93% of their time indoors, there is a growing body of research that is encouraging us to take it outdoors. We all know how good it can feel to be immersed in the natural world, with warm sunlight on our skin, the sound of leaves rustling in the wind, the varying shades of earthy tones and the fragrance of pine needles profoundly calms us and harmonizes our natural rhythms.

For thousands of years, the Japanese culture has been leveraging the stress relieving, anxiety reducing, mood restoring benefits of the forest in a practice called Forest Bathing. Forest bathing is a mindfulness practice of absorbing the beauty of the forest through the senses. Although it can involve exercising, it's mainly focused on simply connecting with the healing power of nature through our senses of sight, hearing, taste, smell and touch.

Researcher Dr. Qing Li says, "Shinrin-yoku is like a bridge. By opening our senses, it bridges the gap between us and the natural world." In his studies, Dr. Li has shown that spending time in the forest lowers stress chemicals and relieves symptoms related to depression, anxiety and attention disorders. Moreover, the more time we spend outside, the more passionate we become about preserving it, which the earth is in desperate need of. Through mindfulness and gratitude for the beauty of nature, we may feel a sense of returning home to ourselves. After all, we're made of the same elements as the stars!

Whether it's an old-growth forest, an urban park, or even a window with a view, nature promotes calm brain wave states and soothes our nervous system. So whenever possible, maximize the few minutes you have to yourself each day by spending them outside!

Student Reflection

What are three ways you could bring more of the outdoors into your life?

1.

_____

2.

_____

3.

_____

We've all been told: "You need to focus!" However, many of us have not been taught how to focus. This is something we can train our minds to do, with practice.

In the movie, The Karate Kid, the sensei taught his student to focus on a single task: waxing a car. The youth was directed to apply the wax with one hand and wipe off the residue with the other. Although it may appear to be a nonessential task, it was directing the young man's attention solely to the job at hand. Later, he applied this focus of mind and body to training in self-defence.

Repeated training using intentional focus helps us to direct our attention amidst the millions of competing external stimuli, such as environmental noises, unrelated thoughts, random scents, etc. (Jha, 2013). By intentionally setting our thoughts on a specific task, we are rewiring neural pathways used for focusing (Kozasa et al., 2011; Lu et al., 2014)

In the following exercise, you will become immersed in your surroundings. Choose an object in nature and consciously focus your attention on that object. Calm your thoughts and let yourself feel connected to your surroundings.

After participating, one Olympic kayaker reported that she frequently focuses intently when kayaking, becoming connected with her environment through directed focus. While in her boat, her paddle is not separate from her, nor is the water. It is all one. The kayaker is the paddle, and the paddle is the water. That is the potential of mindful practice.

Instructions

Setting:

This exercise is best done outdoors, in nature. Ideally, find a natural area nearby, or simply take a walk 2 km around the block.

Exercise:

With the first step, set the intention of becoming completely aware of your surroundings. If you see or hear a bird, intently listen or watch the bird until you almost sense that you are the bird. If the wind blows across your face, feel the wind, sense the wind. If the leaf flutters in the wind, be still and watch its movements until you flow with the leaf.

This may feel bizarre ("how do you become a bird?"). Remind yourself that, a child, you frequently participated in such exercises. you would watch a bird fly or a squirrel climb until you imagined yourself becoming these animals. In our haste to grow up, we lost some of the focusing abilities we had as children. Most people love this exercise because it gives them permission to become that child again.

The objective of this exercise is to observe everything around you. Every time you begin to drift away and lose focus on your surroundings, return to the breath: Observe the breath coming into the nose, down into the belly, and flow back out again. Once you regain your focus on the breath, redirect your focus back to your surroundings. The breath becomes the anchor.

This exercise can be 10 minutes to 45 minutes. Once completed, review the following questions in your journal.

Student Reflection

1. What challenges did you face that hindered your ability to focus on your surroundings?
2. How do they relate to your everyday life?
3. This relates to how we focus in everything
4. Does being peacefully aware of your surroundings help you to remember it more clearly than if you were giving it your usual attentiveness?
5. Did you notice anything new or something that you haven't experienced lately?
6. What is the feeling tone within you, physically, mentally, emotionally and/or spiritually?

Teacher's Note: if time allows, proceed through one of the mindful movement practices with the intention of maintaining this centered, grounded focus.

LESSON 7: THE ART OF EATING MINDFULLY

Note: while this practice is similar to the Raisin Mindfulness Practice below, we left them separate so this one can include a full meal if you wish.

Can you recall a time recently when you frantically shoveled food in your mouth while driving or attending a meeting? While this style of eating has become the norm, studies are warning us that eating on the run contributes to stress-related disorders, digestive issues and obesity.

The ancient yoga tradition affirms these new findings, with its old saying "If you eat standing up, death looks over your shoulder." If we know that eating on the go does not support longevity and wellbeing, how do we break the vicious cycle?

The first step is to acknowledge the value of eating mindfully. When is the last time you stopped to consider that the food you are consuming pumps blood through your heart, nourishes your brain and facilitates the movement of your muscles?

The next step is to give yourself the opportunity to fully devote your attention to the act of eating. It being one of the most important tasks of their day, babies naturally give their complete attention to the act of eating As adults though, we have become so engrossed in the many responsibilities we hold that eating fast food or skipping meals has become commonplace.

Not only does eating mindfully have physical benefits, allowing for greater nutrient absorption (because we actually chew our food), it also engenders a peaceful, calm attitude. Taking that one step further, ancient medical models placed great value on having positive conversation, within a peaceful environment while dining. A blessing before the meal is meant to fill your system with positivity, gratitude and reverence for the creative powers that provided our food.

The following is a guide to a mindful eating exercise:

- Begin by SITTING DOWN and placing your meal in front of you. Hover your hands a few inches over your food or, if it's a snack, hold it in your palm. Close your eyes for a moment and imagine its energy merging with yours, this is the initial step of digesting your food. This is why many traditions today still eat with their hands.

- Contemplate the history of your food before reaching your plate. Where was it grown? Who cared for it? How was it transported?

- Now open your eyes and look at your food, noticing its shape, color and appeal. How do you feel about putting this food in your body? Tune into the rhythm of your breathing, as you anticipate this food becoming part of your whole being.

- Now slowly place a small portion of your meal in your mouth, and without chewing or swallowing right away, move it around with your tongue to explore temperature, texture and taste etc. Take your first bite and notice the initial flavors that burst in your mouth.

- Observe any habitual impulse to devour it quickly and mindfully take the next bite, and the next one. Slow the pace of chewing and chew it more times than you usually would. Let yourself completely experience the act of chewing and tasting your food in this moment.

- Now prepare to swallow, noticing the current texture of the food in your mouth (in Ayurveda, we advise to chew your drink and drink your food☺). Become fully conscious of the act of swallowing, feeling your food slide down into your stomach.

- Take this same approach for each mouthful, staying totally present to the act of eating and digesting. Notice how your body responds to the food while eating it and be aware of signs of fullness (ideally stopping at a 7/10 fullness). Are you eating in response to true hunger or are you eating in reaction to a life situation? We want to eat when we're hungry, not because we're anxious or depressed.
- Instead of setting the bar unrealistically high with intentions of eating each meal this way, you may want to aim to eat one meal a day with mindful awareness. Enjoy!

Teacher's Note: if time allows, proceed through one of the mindful movement practices with the intention of maintaining this centered, grounded focus.

LESSON 8: RAISIN MINDFULNESS PRACTICE

For anyone beginning the path of meditation, it is important to understand the phrase "I do everything with a mind that let's go."

We cling to thoughts and these thoughts in turn become stressors in our lives. All we need to do is let go and for many people, this can be very difficult. These fluctuations of the mind can be likened to a monkey busily jumping on our shoulders.

There is a story about how monkeys are caught in India, using a hollow log with a banana placed inside. The monkey reaches into the log to grab the banana but with a clenched fist cannot remove the item of its desire. The animal remains there, determined to extract the banana from the log, until the trapper comes along and captures the monkey To be free, all the monkey had to do was let go of the banana. We live out the same scenario in our minds, with constant rumination of repetitive thoughts, known to many as 'monkey mind'.

The following mindfulness exercise hones our attention on being fully present to the moment. When we experience present reality, we glimpse freedom. There is an old saying that claims 'The past is gone, the future is imaginary, therefore the present is all that's real.'

Preparation: you will need jumbo organic raisins. Give each member of your class a raisin and ask them to hold it in the palm of their hand Read the following aloud or create your own script using this as a guide.

In your hand, you have a raisin. Take the raisin and roll it between your fingers. Notice the sensation of the raisin in your hand and observe its folds and colors. You may notice a stem still connected to your raisin, where at one time, this stem was the cord that connected the raisin to the plant. The plant was connected to the earth, gleaning nutrients from the sun and soil, which in turn nourished the raisin.

When the raisin had reached its maturity, someone in a far-off part of the world picked it off the vine. They placed it in a crate and shipped it to a factory. The factory then shipped it to a warehouse and the warehouse shipped it to a distributor. The distributor delivered it to the store where I purchased it and brought it to you today. All of these stages required the involvement of many people, and each person has contributed to the energy of this raisin you are now holding.

With the awareness of the many steps it took to land this piece of fruit in your hand, close your eyes and begin to roll the raisin between your fingers. Give yourself a moment to fully experience its texture. What sensations arise?

When you've finished examining the raisin, place it on your tongue, but don't bite it! Using your tongue, roll it around in your mouth. Do you feel its textural variations? Pinch it between your front teeth and gradually allow the teeth to pierce the skin of the raisin, letting its nectar seep into your mouth. You will be tempted to swallow...see if you can withhold to let the sweetness fill your mouth. Continue to chew at least 20 times before swallowing, each bite releasing more and more flavors. Have you ever eaten a simple raisin in this way before?

When you are ready, swallow the raisin As you absorb the raisin into your system, remember that you are connected to the sun, the earth and every person who was involved in the packaging and transportation of this small piece of fruit. Take a moment to enjoy your raisin...

Now open your eyes. You have just experienced what it's like to be totally present to one of the most fundamental, essential life experiences—eating. You did this by maintaining one-pointed focus on a little raisin, free of the common distractions such as technology or conversation.

Teacher's Note: if time allows, proceed through "Mindful Movement practice – Breath Awareness" with the intention of maintaining this centered, grounded focus.

LESSON 9: MOUNTAIN MEDITATION

Introduction

In this day and age with the overload of information and our drive to achieve, many of us are feeling ungrounded and strung out. The Mountain Meditation can provide you with an experience of feeling earthbound, rooted and unwavering, regardless of what is occurring around you.

To find a comfortable seated position, prop your hips up on a block or two or roll up the end of your yoga mat and cross your legs. Resting your back against the wall may also provide further comfort. Rest your hands on your thighs, or, to enhance your concentrate and balance your energy, place your right hand on top of the left, with palms up, thumbs joined. Roll your shoulders back, drop your shoulder blades down your back, open your heart and tuck your chin slightly to align your ears over the shoulders. Imagine your spine as a series of building blocks and adjust your body so that each block creates a solid foundation for the next.

Start to notice your breathing as it enters your body through your nostrils, filling your belly, ribs and chest. Allow it to freely flow out through the nostrils as you exhale. Inhale slowly and deeply, exhale smoothly. As you continue with this rhythm of mindful breathing, imagine your body transforming into a mountain. Your seat becomes the granite base of the mountain, rooting deeply into the earth's center while the tip of your head becomes the peak of the mountain.

As you sit, notice the trees, the flowers, the birds soaring overhead and the small animals running freely over your mountain. All of this activity is happening around you and yet, beneath the surface, the mountain remains the same, rooted deeply into the earth. Nothing moves the mountain.

You soon notice that the days are becoming shorter and the air a little colder. The leaves on the trees begin to change color until they become a bouquet of vibrant oranges, yellows and reds. The entire surface of the mountain is awash with color. The temperature drops and the wind begins to blow blustery chaos over the mountain. Even though the colors and weather patterns change, the mountain remains the same, grounded, unaffected by what is occurring on the surface.

The days become shorter still, the air even crisper. With the rain's force, one by one the leaves start to fall, until finally, only one leaf remains clinging to the tree A strong gust of wind lifts it from the branch, setting it free to float away. This reminds us of the natural process of death and letting go, knowing that these leaves will one day provide nourishment for new life.

The days grow shorter and the first flakes of snow gently fall to the earth. At first, the snowflakes are very large, but as the storm surges, they become smaller and start to whip against the face of the mountain. The winds intensity and brisk temperatures set in.

Snowflakes pound against the rock until the snow almost fully covers the surface of the mountain, making just the tree tops visible. And yet, beneath the snow, the mountain remains the same, rooted and grounded into the earth. Nothing changes the core of the mountain.

As the days progress, the storms diminish and the sun's warmth grows stronger. The days grow longer, slowly melting snow and ice, until the mountain's surface is exposed once again. But beneath the surface of the earth, the mountain remains the same, rooted and unaffected at the center.

As the days grow longer, the warm sun and fallen leaves provide nutrients for plants to sprout up out of the soil, one by one. As the season's change, the buds on the trees burst open and flowers bloom across the mountain range. Once again, a bouquet of color covers the mountain. The animals move freely again over the mountains surface but despite all of this activity, one thing remains the same—the mountain. Grounded, deeply rooted, connected to the center of the earth.

And just as the mountain faces the four seasons, so do you face these four seasons, sometimes within a minute, other times in the span of a day. Regardless of what is sent your way in life, you remain the mountain, unwavering and deeply rooted into the earth.

You are forever the mountain.

Slowly begin to introduce movement into your body, open your eyes and rise to standing. With feet hip width apart, find your mountain pose and establish your roots in this upright position.

Teacher's Note: if time allows, proceed through one of the mindful movement practices with the intention of maintaining this centered, grounded focus.

LESSON 10: GARDEN OF LOVE MEDITATION

Anything you may hold firmly in your imagination can be yours.

William James

There are times in our lives when we feel alone. This feeling of aloneness can turn into a sense of loneliness, which can lead to a belief that we are unlovable. In this visualization we use a process that can help to counter any negative core beliefs about our lovability. We do this by imagining people in our lives who have exhibited unconditional love for us. If we have never felt unconditional love, then we can imagine a pet puppy or bunny providing us with the love we long for. Einstein believed that imagination is one of our most powerful tools because it can create the same emotional response as reality, that's why we love stories so much. Let's work with our imaginations to help free us from the unhelpful feelings of aloneness.

Preparation Stage

Find a quiet place and lie down on your back Adjust yourself until you can rest in a position of comfort. You can use blankets, pillows or other props to help you feel relaxed. If lying on your back is uncomfortable or not possible, shift over to one side or find another position that suits your body.

Exercise

Let's start by focusing on our breath. With each inhalation bring the breath all the way down to the belly, filling the ribcage and then the collarbones. As you exhale, allow yourself to let go and sink deeply into a state of relaxation. With each breath in, we bring life into the body; with each breath out, we let go of anything that separates us from our natural state of being. The breath is like the ocean. The wave flows in and flows out, dispersing any negative emotions into the vastness of the sea. *(let students continue with breath awareness for two minutes).*

Let's imagine now, in your mind's eye, that you are standing in front of a garden gate. Notice the details of the gate, and as you look closer, you see symbols that represent love for you. Walk through the gate and enter into the garden. Look around at all your favourite flowers: roses, daffodils, daisies, who's fragrances uplift you and bring your mind into the present. There is a wonderful state of peace here, one that exists within you at all times. Notice a beautiful fountain in the centre of the garden and walk over to it. The sound of the water is trickling over the stone surface, creating an even deeper sense of tranquility within. As you stand here absorbing the calming sounds and beauty of the garden, you notice a gentle being from far away, approaching you. This is someone in your life, or in your past, who has always been there for you as a source of unconditional love. He or she gradually arrives in front of you and tells you how much you are loved. Your loved one reminds you that you are a gift to the world, so unique and so cherished. Your loved one reminds you that you are not alone and that there is always someone available to help you on your path, you just need to look around, reach out for help and lean into life. With a grateful heart, you tell your loved one how much you appreciate their love and support. Thank them for reminding you that love is always available, which you return to them as well. When you are ready, allow this special being of light to turn and walk away, knowing that you can call on this being anytime you need a boost or reassurance.

When you feel ready, bring your attention back to the sound of the flowing water of the fountain and the fragrance of the flowers. Notice how full your heart is now and turn to walk towards the gate. As you step out of the garden, remind yourself that this unconditional love is yours to receive every step of the way. You are never alone.

Coming back to present moment awareness, slowly introduce movement into your fingers, hands, toes and feet. Roll over onto your side, curl up and take a few easy breaths. This is the foetal position, the time when you lived and grew in your mother's womb, immersed in a pool of love. As a baby, innocent and naturally mindful, you would stare at your hands for hours with awe and wonder for your own heavenly body. This same perspective is your birthright now. As you rise to sitting, come up with a renewed connection to this infinite love and remember that the greatest gift we can give ourselves and others is Love.

Teacher's Note: if time allows, proceed through one of the mindful movement practices with the intention of maintaining this centered, grounded focus.

LESSON 11: MINDFULNESS EXERCISE FOR HARMONIZING INNER AND OUTER ENVIRONMENTS

Sit comfortably, with your hands resting on your thighs or in your lap Let your sit bones root you down into the earth and then feel your spine elongate, reaching upward toward the sky. Invite your breath to become smooth, slow and deep.

Each breath brings you more and more present to the feeling tone within your body in this moment. Take deep and full inhalations, followed by smooth and complete exhalations. As you continue to mindfully breathe here, aware of both the inhalation and the exhalation, see if you can sense a pause at the top of the inhalation, before the breath turns over into the exhalation. Just pause briefly before letting the breath go. Now, at the end of the exhalation, watch for the pause before filling the lungs with oxygen again. Let your body guide this process, as you may be awakening a dormant longing to slow down. Pausing briefly in the moments between the inbreath and outbreath allows us to experience a beautiful inner stillness.

Moving on now, allow your eyes to open and without moving your head or even your eyes, become aware of your outer world—sensing the space around you, the sights, sounds, smells and anything else that catches your attention.

Close your eyes now and turn your attention to your inner landscape—noticing your thoughts, feelings, emotions, sensations and memories as they occur within you.

Now, keeping your eyes closed, expand your awareness to your outer world again, becoming present to the sights, sounds, aromas and temperature around you Feel yourself becoming aware of both your outer world and your inner world—observing with your minds eye the sights, sounds, aromas, and the temperature of your outer world along with the qualities of your inner world, including your thoughts, feelings, body sensations, mental thought forms, memories and images.

Feel the outer world merging with your inner world, the space around you harmonizing with the space within you. Release your ideas of separation and imagine yourself joining with the world around you, you and the whole universe blending into one existence. No barriers, no blockages, just oneness.

> The birds have vanished into the sky
> And now the last cloud drains away.
> We sit together, the mountain and me,
> Until only the mountain remains.
>
> Li Po

As you breathe, you not only breathe *your* body, but the body of the planet. You and the Universe, breathing as one, breathing in unison. You're now one with the expanded, infinite, boundless energy of the whole world.

Return your attention to your body, your breath, sensations within you and the contents of the world around you. Enjoy a few fall out breaths, exhaling deeply with a sigh, letting the feeling of belonging and peace settle deeply within your core. When you're ready, you can inhale, open your eyes and return to the room.

Teacher's Note: if time allows, proceed through one of the mindful movement practices with the intention of maintaining this centered, grounded focus.

LESSON 12: AWAKENING THE FIVE SENSES

Material

- one candle for the center of the room or a candle for each student.
- A tissue with a few drops of peppermint essential oil for each student.
- A tissue with a few drops of lavender oil for each student.
- A food sample such as a grape, orange slice or dark chocolate chip

If you are able to do this exercise outside, do so, otherwise, find music that emphasizes the sounds of nature, especially bird's songs.

Introduction

So much of our waking hours today are spent in sensory overload, a state in which our senses are bombarded with too much information for our systems to tolerate and make sense of Too much sensory stimulation, where an excessive amount of information is entering our lives through the senses leads to distress and imbalance.

We can, however, be more proactive by monitoring how much information we consume as well as the quality of information that reaches our nervous systems. The information we consume through our senses can heal and calm, uplift and inspire us, or conversely, drain and damage, distort and depress us. What's more, information that we absorb through the senses, such as images, or sounds, can linger in our memories forever. That said, it is essential that we become discerning and selective with regards to the sensory stimuli we are exposed to.

One of the most healing practices we can do for our health and longevity is to intentionally nourish our senses with peaceful, beautiful experiences. We can best do this by surrounding ourselves in nature, whether it's a forest, a stream, an ocean, a city park, an atrium, whatever you can find in the moment.

The following exercise is designed to nourish your senses, in turn soothing and balancing the systems of your body and mind. The imagination is extremely powerful so for simplicity and convenience, we will visualize ourselves amidst the elements of nature so that we can do this anytime, anywhere.

Sitting comfortably, take a few moments to relax your body and settle your breathing.

Let's begin our exercise of nourishing the senses by lighting our candle. With so many negative, violent images that we are exposed to every day, it is important to take time to feed our sight with images that calm us. As you light your candle, notice the wick quickly turn to fire and watch the flame flicker with aliveness. Notice the wax melting softly and the objects around the flame glowing in its presence. Breathing deeply and slowly, observe any changes in the feeling tone of your body as you simply focus on the candle and its flame.

Next, we'll shift our attention to our sense of hearing. Sound has a big impact on our nervous system. Let's imagine or literally invite the melodic sound of birds to enter the space within our minds. Follow the song of the birds, and let their sound fill your inner ear. Breathing softly here and notice how the music of nature affects the way you feel.

Next, we'll turn our focus to the sense of smell, known to have the most immediate effect on the body and brain. Knowing this, we can use the sense of smell to enhance our wellbeing and awaken our spirits. Lift the tissue with the essential oil of peppermint and observe the way it affects your system. How does it feel passing through your nasal passage? Are you experiencing peppermint's uplifting and cooling properties? Next, lift the tissue with lavender oil and notice how you feel with this aroma entering your system. Can you sense lavender's calming, soothing properties? Is there a particular smell for you that awakens a sense of wellbeing, comfort and safety? Perhaps the smell of cooking, baking, fresh picked flowers or bubble bath? Can you infuse your life with this fragrance more often to elicit these positive feelings?

Next, let's explore the enjoyable sense of taste, the sense that has lasting effects on our body. So much so that we often carry memories of what we ate as children well into adulthood. Taste is one of the ways in which we attempt to soothe our overloaded systems, but unfortunately many of the foods of convenience today actually deplete our health instead of restoring it. A naturally sweet, delicious tasting food in ancient medicine is said to make the mouth happy and calm. Take whatever food choice is provided here and place it in your hand, letting the first stages of digestion and absorption begin here. Become aware of its texture, shape, size and color. Then place the piece of food on your tongue and let the enzymes in your mouth dissolve it slowly. As you swallow, notice how your body receives this food, does it appeal to your stomach? If we ate with this level of awareness all the time, we would be able to identify foods that give us life and foods that drain us.

Finally, let's examine the effects of touch on our systems. The entire human body is a network of sensitive touch receptors, and therefore everything it comes into contact with elicits a reaction of some kind within us. Take a moment to become aware of the clothes you're wearing and how they feel on your skin. What about your shoes, hair accessories, glasses, or a hat? What feedback is your body giving you about these items that are touching your skin? Now slowly, mindfully bring your fingertips to touch each other, hand to hand and notice the sensations this awakens Now place your middle fingers just on the outside of the nostrils and observe how it feels to gently touch your face. Proceed to sliding your hands up your face, over your head, and down your neck, continuing in this circular motion a few times to give yourself a brief massage. How does it feel to touch yourself so mindfully and tenderly?

Let's stand up and form a line, one in front of the other. Now, with the intent to exchange healing touch, rest your hands on the person's shoulders in front of you and take a few quiet, deep breaths. Notice how this basic gesture of both giving and receiving contact on the shoulders affects the way you feel. You can slowly begin to squeeze the person's neck muscles with the pads of your thumbs and fingers. Exhaling with a loud haaaa is a great way to complement the relaxation response that this massage usually brings. After two minutes or so, each person can turn and switch directions, massaging the person who was behind them for two minutes. When complete, thank your classmates and return to your seat.

Debrief: how do you feel now? More awake, more present, more sensitive? More connected? If you feel more agitated or disconnected, this may be a sign that there is some inner healing to do with the assistance of a therapist.

If this exercise was positive, how and where can you apply this practice of sensory mindfulness into your daily life?

Teacher's Note: if time allows, proceed through one of the mindful movement practices with the intention of maintaining this centered, grounded focus.

LESSON 13: MINDFUL COMMUNICATION IN PARTNERS

Leading with awareness of the self and non-judgmental listening, let's agree that what is shared here remains between the two of you, and not discussed outside of the partnering exercise unless you both desire to. Let's also agree to be present without distractions, like checking your phone.

The following exercises foster open expression within a safe, supportive environment while teaching students how to truly listen for what the person is saying and what their needs are. We live in a world of noise—everyone is talking, no one is listening so this may feel quite foreign!

Giving someone your full attention as she speaks may feel unusual and even awkward at first, and that's okay. Anything we do for the first time often is. Try to stay with it however, because enhancing your communication skills, in particular your listening skills, can benefit every area of your life!

Exercise 1

In this exercise, partner A chooses to share first while partner B agrees to do the listening. Partner A begins by speaking for five minutes on a topic of interest, a pressing issue, or anything at all. Her job is to be mindful of the words she uses, the content she speaks about and the tone by which she says it. She attempts to say what she wants with as much accuracy as possible. The speaker has permission to pause, to take a breath and to feel, so that she can speak from a place of truth.

Partner B, as the listener, responds by staying on topic with the speaker, not relating the conversation to her own similar experience. She can verbally respond by asking questions or offering encouragement. Keeping in mind that 80% of our communication occurs beyond our verbal language, she can also non-verbally respond, through body language, eye contact and other displays of interest and engagement.

After this first round, partners can switch roles and then take five minutes to debrief and discuss the experience.

Questions for Inquiry

Did this type of communication feel different from what you're used to? If so, how?
  Did you feel heard?
  Were you more aware of the words you spoke?
  How do you feel after this brief experiment in mindful communication?
  What benefits can you imagine might come from being more present in your day to day conversations?

Exercise 2

This next exercise increases the difficulty, and perhaps the discomfort as partner A, the speaker, talks freely for five minutes again about that which is relevant or important in her life, with the same degree of mindful awareness.

Partner B this time sits comfortably and listens attentively and reverently but without verbal feedback. She simply holds a compassionate presence without the distraction of words.

The listener solely communicates non-verbally with affirmative body language like nodding the head or using facial expressions. This will likely feel very awkward and that's okay, just keep going.

When the time is up, partner B takes one minute to mirror back what partner A said, in as much verbatim as possible, using the speaker's language.

When it's time, partners can switch roles, allowing partner B to speak for five minutes, while partner A assumes the listening role, practicing non-verbal communication and fully listening for what the person is truly saying.

Questions for Inquiry

Describe your experience of sharing in a state of open, undistracted presence?

What did you discover about yourself and about communication in general through this type of communication?

How did you feel during and after this exercise?

What benefits can you see would come from practicing this depth of listening in your day to day communication?

Unhealthy communication breeds disharmony, stress, frustration and emotional distance. Healthy communication on the other hand, fosters self-worth and creates deep connections, intimacy and happiness!

Teacher's Note: if time allows, proceed through one of the mindful movement practices with the intention of maintaining this centered, grounded focus.

LESSON 14: WEST AFRICAN DJEMBE DRUMMING AS A MINDFULNESS PRACTICE

By Krishinda McBride

"The rhythm is in your blood" is an African proverb that resonates from the beat of the drum. Within the African diaspora, the drum represents more than a mere musical instrument. It is emblematic in its connections to the spirit, culture and history of African descent people. The beginnings of African history and culture are documented through oral stories and images. Information on one of best-known drums from West Africa, the djembe (pronounced 'jem-beh') is rich and as diverse as the individuals within the African Diaspora. The djembe is shaped like a large goblet and played with bare hands.

Given the oral sharing of stories and traditions the legends and/ or origins of the djembe are varied The djembe is believed to have originated around 1300 A.D. with the "Numu" social class of professional blacksmith from the Mandinka (or Maninke) people of Western Africa. The Numu played the instrument during the smelting of iron ore and are the first people to be associated with the djembe. Historians believe that when the Numu blacksmiths migrated, the drum and its culture spread through West Africa. According to Mandinka legend, the djembe is said to have come about through a genie (known as a djinn) that gifted the tree to a Mandinka blacksmith and taught them how to carve it into a djembe.

The most commonly told story about the djembe is that a villager's wife was pounding grain in her mortar one day when she pounded through the bottom. Her husband happened to be in the vicinity with a goat skin, which they stretched over the hole in the mortar to make the very first djembe. The term "djembe" originates from a saying by the Bambara people in Mali "Anke djé, anke bé" which translates to "everyone gather together in peace". The saying also defines the drums purpose. *According to the Malinke people a skilled drummer is one who "can make the djembe talk", meaning that "the player can tell an emotional story."*

In West African society, certain instruments such as the ngoni, balafon and the kora are known to have heredity restrictions, meaning that they may only be played by members of the griot (storyteller/historian) caste The djembe is not a griot instrument and today there are no restrictions on who may become a "djembefola" (one who plays the djembe). The djembe is primarily the instrument used at marriages, baptisms, funerals and celebrations. The djembe is central to the musical heritage of West Africa. The djembe is also harmonious in its interaction of communications between drums, communities and individuals.

Mindfulness & the Djembe

> Mindfulness means paying attention in a particular way; on purpose, in the present moment and non-judgementally
>
> Jon Kabat-Zinn

The process of playing or interacting with the djembe causes an individual to pay attention in a particular way. The djembefola purpose is to focus in the moment. In making connections to mindfulness, when one plays the djembe they are focused on the present for purposeful play (marriage celebration, birth of a child, harvesting, etc.). Drumming with a djembe hand drum creates a physical connection between the individual and the natural environment through the goat skin while simultaneously producing sound and rhythm. The djembe's connection to mindfulness is evident when you play the instrument, and direct attention, on purpose, to the rhythm of your hands on the drum, while being fully present in the moment to the sound they are creating.

Playing the djembe has meditative and positive social qualities. When a djembefola begins to connect and synchronise breathing to the rhythm and movement of their drum, a rhythmic groove is developed. This rhythmic groove within the djembe player can be defined as a journey of self-expression and self- identification. A djembe player's rhythmic groove is their voice of communication and empowerment. Djembe players trust their rhythms and grooves as they play. There are some traditional beats, but like the oral history within the African diaspora, information and rhythms may vary from region to region and from djembefola to djembefola.

Playing the djembe cultivates nonjudgement, patience, an open mind and trust in oneself to let go while still being present in the moment of drumming. Djembe drumming has shown to have positive physical, social and emotional outlets for students. Djembe drumming is also being reported today as providing a "true circle of life" due to its positive effects on an individual's health. There is strong evidence of the therapeutic potential for drumming in a group, showing significant social and emotional improvement. (Bittman, 2001; Smith, Viljoen, McGeachie ,2014).

Curriculum Connections

In making connection to the djembe and the P-12 educational curriculum, the following areas of need are examined: social, communication, emotional and cognitive.

- **Social Needs:** The djembe provides an avenue to focus and connect with others in a satisfying way. Drumming is a collaborative and interactive process. Participating in a drumming experience can develop skills such as self-awareness, turn-taking and sharing, as well as assist individuals in feeling that they are part of a group and contributing to a group process.
- **Communication Needs:** Playing the djembe can be a useful way to communicate nonverbally and to "listen" to another person's nonverbal communication.
- Fine and Gross Motor Skills. This may almost seem self-evident, but different playing techniques can be used to help work on different fine and gross motor skills. The coordination of breath and movement with repetitive rhythm has a physiological calming effect on an individual.
- **Emotional Needs:** The playing of the djembe can be a valuable channel for the release of intense emotions; drumming can assist in rebuilding a sense of efficacy and self-worth. Playing the djembe develops inward awareness as well as outward attentiveness. Playing the djembe also fosters self-control, patience and cooperation.
- **Cognitive Needs:** By participating in a drumming experience, individuals can work on attention, impulse control, decision-making skills and patience. Djembe drumming can build valuable skills for processing and communicating information while also developing skills for channeling intense emotions and impulses into a creative positive activity.

Djembe drumming can foster and be part of a positive culturally responsive pedagogy strategy When an educator uses the medium of the djembe drum to validate, affirm and build bridges with their students, they are fostering a community of learning through the development of relationships. The djembe provides a positive avenue for individuals to let go and find their rhythmic groove of expression and empowerment. Although the djembe has ancestral ties to West Africa, it is an instrument that invites "everyone to gather together in peace".

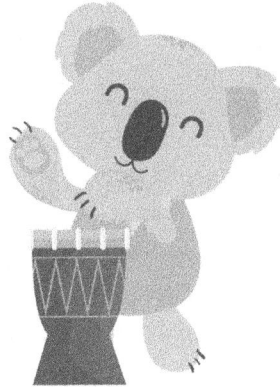

LESSON 15: BODY TALK

The human body is one of the most ingenious machines on the planet, capable of performing hundreds of automatic metabolic processes. Your body is able to attack incoming pathogens, digest food, watch TV and secrete the right hormone in just the right amount, all at the same time! With over 100,000 diseases that the body is susceptible to, it is nothing short of a miracle that our bodies function as well as they do, so often with no support from us!

Even though we are the most evolved and conscious creatures on the planet, it is a common habit amongst us humans to overlook our body's needs, focusing instead on our life goals, entertainment, socialization and of course, indulging the senses.

We push our bodies to the point of pain through exercise, or we don't give it enough activity, we under eat, we over eat, we consume foods and substances that intoxicate our bodies, and we all too often exhaust it through insufficient sleep.

We alienate our bodies from our day to day life experience…we disassociate from parts of the body that hold unfavorable memories…we numb sensations and override our body's messages with prescription drugs, sugar, caffeine and alcohol so we don't have to listen to its requests.

Our society today profits on self-hatred and body dissatisfaction, and so we're encouraged to criticize and condemn our bodies.

We can be cruel to our bodies, not because we don't care, but because don't know how to love and accept our bodies. Society teaches us to strive for unrealistic standards of perfection and that hating the body is somehow productive. But nothing good has ever come out of criticism and scorn.

All of this hatred and rejection of the body has a powerful energetic effect -- dis-eased thinking of the mind leads to dis-eased states within the body. And we all know deep down, that poor health brings suffering, not happiness. Our health therefore, is the foundation for every other aspect of our lives.

When we believe we're inadequate, when we feel pressured to be something different than what we are, the fight or flight response in our NS turns on, causing us to feel constantly on edge as we live in a state of hyper arousal and self-protection. Fighting against our bodies all the time creates a battlefield within our inner landscape, which brings mind/body disharmony and emotional anguish.

Despite the fact that many of us mistreat our bodies and put them through so much pain and abuse, our bodies remain loyal and hard working. The change however, does not need to occur in our bodies. In order to experience lasting health and inner peace, the change must occur within our minds. When we change our minds about the miraculous machine we call the body, we shift from living on a battlefield, to living in thanksgiving. We shift from being dis-embodied, living outside of ourselves, to becoming embodied beings, where we actually take up residence within our bodies and heal our number one relationship.

You may be asking—how can I love my body when it causes me so much frustration and anger? Consider the possibility that your body is not at fault, society is. Consider that there is nothing you need to change about your body in order to love it…imagine giving yourself permission to love and accept your body just as it is, in all its uniqueness. How might that feel? Perhaps settled, free, peaceful, relaxed. This feeling of calm is the result of harmonizing your mind with your body, which is our intent for this meditation.

It is possible to turn the wheel on the momentum of body hatred and the first step is the practice of acceptance and gratitude. It is a practice, because it may not feel natural or authentic initially, and that's okay. We're simply unlearning the faulty beliefs we've been taught for many years.

Let's start by taking a few deep, cleansing breaths. In through the nose, out through the mouth. In through the nose, out with a sign. One more time, breathing in fully, breathing out completely.

Moving on to a brief body scan, you are invited to be present to your body with a neutral attitude, without judgment. You may not be able to send it appreciation but at least withhold criticism for the next few moments.

Continue to notice your breathing and follow its rhythm in and out of your body.

Inhale and visualize your inner landscape expanding, exhale and allow your muscular network to relax deeply. As we move through the various aspects of our being, maintain a smooth and steady breathing pattern, allowing your body to relax.

Turn your attention to your head and your scalp and notice how you're holding your head, your face, your jaw...

Drop your attention to your throat, your neck, chest and shoulders... just notice what there is to notice about these parts of your body with an attitude of curiosity.

Scan down now into your belly, your pelvis, and along your back...what information is available to you here?

Drawing your attention to your legs, your knees, your calves, your feet and even your toes. Notice how you're holding your lower body...remember, we're not here to judge, we're not here to fix anything, we're just noticing what is.

Become fully aware of your whole internal space, noticing sensations in your body, including those that are pleasant and those that may be causing you discomfort or even pain. Just observe.

Take a few more slow, deep wavelike breaths and invite yourself open to a new way of thinking and a healthier way of relating to your body.

Let's move on now to communicating with the body.

With the intention of making peace and building trust with all aspects of yourself, ask yourself if there is anything you want to say to your body? Take a moment to share it now...

Just imagine, what does your body have to say in response? Listen attentively, like you would to a dear friend.

Continue this dialogue for a few more moments...breathing smoothly and deeply.

Paying attention to your body, is there an area calling out for your attention?

What does it want to tell you? What does it need?

Thank this part of your body for communicating. You may feel ready to reassure your body that you will listen more attentively in the future.

Imagine your mind and body joining, like two sailors working together to propel their boat in a common direction.

Let's practice gratitude now, giving thanks for the body you have been given. Not the body you could have if you worked out a few more hours a week, not the body you might have if you got this or that cosmetic surgery, but your body as it is, right now. Explore the possibility of being unconditional with your body.

Your health and wellbeing are worth it. Your body is most deserving of your own care and compassion right now. Consider giving to yourself the same love you give to others.

Is there a part of your body that you can offer some appreciation to? Just choose one body part and extend your gratitude to it for what it allows you to do and enjoy.

Acknowledge yourself for extending this gratitude to your body. This is the first step in making peace with yourself.

Writing Assignment

If you were to write a letter to your body, what might you say to it?
Sample letter:

Dear body,

Today I choose to work with you and move toward health and healing.

I know our relationship has been difficult and we've both struggled. Sometimes life isn't easy and living in opposition with you makes it even harder. I've not always treated you as well as I could have and I've often put my own needs and desires above yours. I apologize for that.

I've ignored your messages and you may have lost trust in me. I've felt so much frustration and disappointment with you, and I now realize how hard you've worked to keep up.

I am learning to understand the ways in which you communicate. I know that illness and injury are some of the ways you attempt to spark my attention.

I am ready to listen to you now and I am appreciative of our connection. No longer is there a you and a me separation, but a 'we', working together and living in harmony from now on.

I commit to being present to your needs as you grow and change because I recognize how important you are to my existence. You are the vessel that allows me to experience life in human form and with that awareness, I now treat you with more respect.

Thank you, body,
Signed: _____

Next step: if your body were to write you a letter, what would it say? Simply listen for the answer and write freely.

LESSON 16: MINDFULNESS AND FORGIVENESS

Life is a wonderful gift and the mindfulness practices included in this manual, such as positivity and gratitude, can certainly help us to stay on the sunny side of life through all its ups and downs. Sometimes, however, we have very difficult life experiences that cause us to fall into deep states of suffering. It's at these times, when our sense of security and peace of mind are replaced with confusion and sorrow, that we can turn to the powerful practice of forgiveness.

Remember that no one is ever loyal and loving all the time. People can become so consumed in their own needs that they do harmful things to others. And despite our deepest commitments to treat people with respect, we can still mess up ourselves and make mistakes, hurting others—even the one's we love most.

That's why forgiveness is a fundamental, basic practice for being human, which all spiritual and religious traditions point to as a path for freedom and peace. Indeed, we have a great capacity for tenderness and love. But many of us over time, become buried beneath layers of pain, resentment and hatred. Without forgiveness, we can end up like the classic scrooge character, emotionally stunted, distrusting of others and deceitful.

It's easy to imagine life without forgiveness though, because we see it in the media every day. Hostile behavior is demonstrated in politics, and destructive, manipulative leadership is endorsed by society. Violence is still promoted in many sporting arenas and vengeance is the main theme of action films today. What this teaches us is how to carry around the pain of the past, reinforcing the pattern of harmful feelings over and over again.

Just look at the cultural battles happening around the world today. People are taking passionate stances against others and justifying violent behavior, which only spills pain onto the canvas of family's lives, passing resentments down through generations. But we don't have to carry these burdens of the past. It is possible to let go of pain and trauma and, according to Sarah Montana, it's the only true path to personal freedom. After a troubled teen murdered her brother and mother in their home, she suffered for years with all-consuming hatred and grief. Eventually, she came to the realization that she had to let go of her grievance with her family's killer in order to experience any semblance of peace in her life. Her Ted Talk is well worth the watch: *The Real Risk of Forgiveness–And Why It's Worth It.*

Sarah would most likely agree with Jack Kornfield's statement "To carry hatred and resentment is to volunteer for suffering", but to practice forgiveness is to let go of past grievances and stop wishing harm onto others.

Stories of forgiveness remind us of the healing potential that lies within the human heart. Victor Frankl, Nazi prison camp survivor, teaches us that no matter who we are, emotional freedom is possible. "We who lived in the concentration camps, can remember those of us who walked through the huts, comforting others and giving away their last morsels of bread crumbs. They may have been few in number, but they offer sufficient proof that everything can be taken from us, but the last of our human freedoms is the freedom to choose our attitude in any given circumstance", says Frankl. After losing his wife and family in Auschwitz, Victor went on to contribute great things to humanity, because he was able to forgive and out of his brokenness, create beauty.

If you've not been hurt or betrayed yet, you likely will be in some way throughout the course of your lifetime. And when you do experience the pain of abandonment or perhaps abuse, you will know that the only true path of peace is to take the road of forgiveness. But if we don't understand what forgiveness really is, we might resist it, assuming it's a process of condoning another's harmful behavior, but it's not. To forgive is not to say "Oh, no worries, it's alright" In Sarah's words, "When you say 'I forgive you', what you're really saying is, 'I know what you did is not okay but I recognize that you are more than that. I don't want to hold us captive to this anymore. I can heal myself and I don't need anything from you.'"

Forgiveness is not a quick fix, however. Depending on the pain we carry, we can't typically just press the delete button and feel good again. It may require repeated practice that acknowledges our pain and sorrow before we are ready to let go and experience emotional freedom. It's more than just *going* through the pain, it's about *growing* through the pain of the past.

In today's world, we have replaced the difficult but rewarding work of forgiveness with numbing agents like entertainment, busy-ness, pills, substances and sugar. While this may pacify the pain temporarily, over time it creates an imbalance in our system, causing even more pain. We need to give ourselves time and space to express our sadness or anger in a way that harms no one, including ourselves. If we don't *grow* through the pain, and attempt to simply *go* through it, we only end up building armor which can successfully block the pain but can create barriers to the goodness as well. Makes you wonder about the 'Under Armour' brand that's become so popular these days!

Martin Luther King described forgiveness as a soul force, because it requires more than just will alone, it's an effort that must come from the deepest part of our being. The parents of the victims of the Humbolt Hockey team tragedy have exercised great *soul force* by showing mercy and compassion to the truck driver who hit their bus and destroyed so many lives.

Similarly, just a few days after her daughter Rehteah committed suicide after years of cyber bullying, Leah Parsons advised enraged friends and family at a vigil to protest for peace and justice, not revenge. As we expand our awareness to the possibilities for peace inherent within forgiveness, we find real-life examples of devastating heart break and heroic acts of forgiveness that inspire us to do the same.

Why do we forgive anyway? Because we must in order to have any hope for peace in our future. Our forgiveness work may be directed at ourselves, for things we've done in the past that we regret. Admitting that we have hurt others is a powerful way of reminding ourselves that everyone makes mistakes. We're all doing the best we can with the skills we have in the moment.

Our forgiveness work can be directed toward another person as well, but we're not doing this for others, we're doing this for our own healing. After all, the other person may not be in misery at all, in fact, they might very well have forgotten all about you. We're the ones suffering, so we're the ones with the work to do.

Let's be clear that the person we are forgiving need not be present in our lives to do this work, especially if they are emotionally or physically unsafe to be around. True forgiveness work is based on willingness to release the pain in our heart without doing further harm. This is why Gandhi called forgiveness an act of bravery. The true heroes in our world are those who can forgive, knowing that hatred brings pain and love brings healing.

Hatred never ceases by hatred, but by love alone is healed.

Dhamapada

Student Reflection

Think of the most generous hearted, compassionate person you know. How do they respond to change, difficulty and loss?

What burdens of resentment are you carrying? Can you imagine life without that heavy weight?

Do a research project on the proven benefits of forgiveness on one's mental and physical health.

How can we forgive? The following are two practices for forgiveness to do with your class, depending on their readiness:

Entering the Forest of Forgiveness

Settle into a comfortable seat and imagine before you a footpath into the forest. With your left or right foot, step onto the forest floor. With each step, as you lift your back foot, you let go of the outside world and step deeper into the forest of forgiveness. Continuing to walk along this path, you notice sunlight shining through the trees, almost like a spotlight guiding you on your way. Notice the flowers, the trees, the birds all around you, contributing to the peace and serenity of this place.

In the distance you hear a roaring sound, you're not sure what it is but as you come around a corner, you see a raging waterfall cascading into a beautiful blue pool of water below. You come to the edge of the waterfall and listen to its roar You're so close that you can feel the mist caressing your skin, cleansing you of all fear, sadness, and resentment. The cleansing spray brings you into a deeply peaceful state.

After standing for a few moments letting the water wash over you, you turn around and see someone walking toward you. This is someone who you have harbored resentment or anger toward, someone living or dead, it may even be your past self. Allow them to approach you, watching them stop a safe distance away As they stand before you, share the grievance that you have between you. Picture saying to them, "It no longer serves me to hold onto this resentment and anger, in my mind, body or heart. Therefore, I now let go of these feelings and the past and extend forgiveness to you." See the other person accept your forgiveness and bow slightly in agreement.

When you feel complete, visualize this person turning to walk back into the forest, and watch them disappear. As they do, imagine reciting once again "I release you and I free myself from the pain of the past." You then turn to focus on the purifying energy of the waterfall, allowing the mist to wash over you again.

After a few moments, you find your path and begin your journey back through the forest. You notice a new lightness of being and a joy in your heart. Just as it did on your way in, the sun continues to shine through the trees, leading you back to the entrance where you first began your journey through the forest of forgiveness.

Arriving at the edge of the path, one foot steps back into the world as the back foot releases the past one last time. Returning your attention to your breathing body in the here and now, take a few moments to adjust to your new reality before slowly opening your eyes and returning to the moment. Peace, peace, peace.

The Forgiveness Practice

The following is a structure of forgiveness, given to us from the Buddhist tradition. It is designed to soften and humble the heart by starting with the mistakes we've made first, priming us for the act of forgiving another.

1. Find a quiet seat and tune into your breathing. In a quiet, settled state, reflect on a time in your life when you knowingly or unknowingly harmed, betrayed or abandoned someone. Offer yourself forgiveness and let go of any guilt or shame you may be carrying from that experience.

2. Reflect on a time in your past when you have hurt or harmed yourself, perhaps by letting a boundary be crossed, or failing to defend yourself or inflicting injury on yourself in some way. Offer your past-self forgiveness now, reassuring yourself that you were doing your best to take care of yourself with the skills you had at the time.

3. Consider a time in your life when someone else wounded you in some way, emotionally or physically. Take a few gentle breaths here and offer them forgiveness to the degree that you can at this time. Imagine the energetic chords of connection being cut, setting you free and releasing the other person. Relax your body, breathe deeply and applaud yourself for doing such important and brave work.

Note that it's helpful to practice forgiveness with small things so that when/if something big happens, it is a practiced skill that you can draw upon. Life is uncertain, people are imperfect, and forgiveness is an excellent tool for helping us release pain so that we can enjoy our lives.

Pillar 2
Movement Practices

These mindful movement sequences are designed to awaken our awareness of the body and breath. These postures, or body forms, restore health and harmony of every system in the body, build muscular strength and flexibility and bring about a sense of deep calm. Given that the body is connected to the breath, the breath is connected to the mind and the mind is connected to our emotions, as we influence our body through this movement practice, we also impact our whole being.

In our mindful movement practice, we are not attempting to break personal best records for flexibility or strength, although that may happen as a result of regular practice. What we are aiming for is to simply place our full attention on our breathing, our body and the sensations that various postures illicit. As you move, notice how your breath changes as you flow through different postures. How does your breath respond to the easy ones? How does your breathing change in the more challenging ones? As you move, become curious about your body in a non-judgmental way. Are there postures that reveal deep tension you've not noticed before? Are there postures that demonstrate your strength? As you move, notice the various types of sensation in your body. What are you feeling in this shape? Is it stretchy, tingly or tight? Does the inbreath and outbreath bring different sensations? What about your emotional reaction to a posture—do you notice pride, embarrassment, frustration or peace arise?

This mental state of neutral awareness with the absence of rejection, expectation or criticism invites us to just be. It is here where tension seems to naturally dissolve. Another term for mindfulness is remembering, where we return home to our natural state of present moment awareness, without all the conditioned standards imposed on us by society. May this practice of mindful movement be a process of remembering, that reunites the many aspects of yourself into a unified, integrated whole.

TERMS

Taking your Baseline	the practice of drawing your awareness to the feeling tone in your body in the moment.
Growing Edge	your growing edge is the green zone of your movement practice, where you're challenged but not in pain.
Asana	a body shape designed to stretch and strengthen.
Pranayama	the practice of applying breathing techniques.
Savasana	lying on one's back in stillness for a period of time, with the intent to deeply relax, heal the body and quiet the mind.

THE GRIP: A NOTE TO ALL OWNERS OF BODIES

Ever sit and notice how you're holding your body in any given moment? In yoga and meditation, we learn to relax the body by refining the flow of the breath. The idea behind yoga and especially pranayama (the practice of directing the breath) is to bring the breath into a smooth rhythm which serves to calm our thoughts and release deep-seated tension.

Richard Rosen describes a component of our lives that can delay this experience of quieting the mind, which he calls the grip. The grip is a collection of physical tension that tends to live in one main area of the body, which is unique for all of us depending on our life experiences, stress levels etc.

He believes the grip to be a representation of our small self, showing up in our bodies. The small self is similar to what people in the west refer to as ego, the aspect of ourselves that tries to convince us that we are separate from others while encouraging us to judge and criticize to widen the gap. Not only does the grip attempt to protect us from the terrors of outside world, but it also serves to protect the outside world from the (perceived) terrors inside of us.

We all have our own unique storage cell of tension, for some it's in the belly, for others it's in the neck and for many it's found in the head. Wherever the grip exists in your body, chances are it developed for good purpose. One client who was physically abused as a child and told that she was never going to amount to anything because she was female carries her tension in her lower abdomen, ironically in her womb.

The grip is very clever. The trouble with this protective mechanism is that where there is tension, or pain, there is no energy flow. Where there is no energy flow, there is no life. Discovering the location of your own unique grip and consciously softening to allow energy to re-awaken that area, encourages life to flow again, and hence wards of atrophy and disease.

By incorporating movement into our mindfulness practice, we can alter deep tension patterns and create a more peaceful inner environment within which to live our lives.

MOVEMENT SITTING COMBINATION CLASS

Most people, including and especially children, have a difficult time doing a sitting practice in the beginning of the mindfulness journey, therefore, it is helpful to incorporate movement into the experience. Infusing stillness with periods of movement is also very helpful for trauma survivors who are striving to stay within their window of tolerance.

It is recommended to start with a short centering sitting practice (on the floor or a chair) and then move to gentle asanas or walking (see walking practices in this movement section). Each segment of the practice can last between five to seven minutes (perhaps shorter for younger grades) and the transition can be noted by sounding a singing bowl or calming bells.

The following is an example of a twenty-minute combination practice:

FIRST SITTING SESSION—INTRODUCTION

Let's begin our practice by finding a comfortable seat in a chair. Rest your feet on the floor, place your hands in your lap, align your spine, soften your belly, lift your heart and relax your face.

With eyes closed or slightly open gazing down, moving onto circle breathing now, where we breathe in and up along one side of the circle and breathe out and down along the other side of the circle. Smooth, deep and full inbreaths, followed by smooth, soft and steady outbreaths. Let's use the breath as an anchor for our minds to return to, by silently repeating "Breathing in, breathing out."

You may find yourself becoming distracted at the top of the circle, between inbreath and outbreath or at the bottom, between the outbreath and the inbreath, but that's okay because we have the ability to witness our mind being present and to also notice when we've become distracted, which enables us to return to the moment over and over again.

Breathing in, breathing out, breathing in, breathing out.

Notice your body relax as you simply rest in the moment here, nothing to do, nowhere to go, this time is allotted for practice and this practice alone. Reassure yourself that your responsibilities will be waiting for you when you're finished, and you'll be better able to do your work having done this practice. So just relax and savor this moment.

Teacher rings the bell and invites students to quietly rise to standing and spread out so they have room to move.

FIRST STANDING ARM FLOW

Let's begin with a simple arm flow by inhaling arms out to the sides and up overhead, exhale palms together and slide them down the midline of your body. Again, inhale arms up, exhale hands down the center of your body. Keep going, keep flowing, at a slow and mindful pace. Notice the sensations through your shoulder joint as the arms move through their range of motion.

See if you can coordinate the beginning, middle and end of your breath with the beginning, middle and end of the movement so that each movement is filled with the breath, without holding the breath at any point. Relax your face and enjoy this feeling of harmonizing your breath with your movements. Stay rooted through your feet as your upper body flows. Remember your anchor words "Breathing in, breathing out."

Teacher rings the bell and invites students to sit again, settling into a comfortable position that allows them to be still for a few minutes.

SECOND SITTING SESSION

Return your awareness to proper posture, feet grounded, hands resting, belly soft and spine aligned. With eyes closed or slightly open gazing down, tune into your breathing once again, breathing in, breathing out. Focusing on just one thing for a period of time is hard work, so this time, let's identify a spot in your body to help our minds stay present. You can choose a part of your body where you feel the breath flowing in and out, like the nostrils, or the chest or the belly. Settle on one spot in your body to help anchor your attention and focus on any sensations and movement there.

The neat thing about focusing on our breath is that every breath is new and different in some way from the last one, so pay full attention to each breath as it arises, as though you're discovering something for the first time, (because you are). Feel the sensations in the spot where your breath flows, noting the cool air entering the nostrils on the inbreath, the hot air leaving the nostrils on the outbreath, the expansion of the belly and chest on the inhalation, and the contraction of the chest and belly on the exhalation. The breath is always right under your nose, there to help calm and relax you anytime you need it.

Teacher rings the bell and invites students to quietly rise to standing and spread out, so they have room to move.

SECOND STANDING FLOW

Let's repeat the movement sequence we did last time, inhaling arms out and up, exhaling palms together as they slide down the center of your body. Do this a few times, remaining aware of your breath filling out the full spectrum of your movements.

When you're ready, inhale arms overhead and exhale add a forward fold by letting your torso follow your hands toward the earth. Linger here in a gentle forward fold for two or three breaths, dangling the arms and head like seaweed. Let the inhalation lift you up, uncurling the spine vertebrae by vertebrae, lifting your head last and reaching your arms to the sky. Let the exhalation release your upper body downward, folding at the hips, bending your knees if you need to. Inhale gently rise up, gradually stacking your spine and reaching tall, exhale slide hands down center and fold. Continue with this flow, moving slowly and mindfully.

Notice the new sensations through the legs and backside and the strength of your core that's required to rise slowly back up. Feel free to add a slight smile as you flow, reflecting the inner gratitude you have for the body you've been given.

Teacher rings the bell and invites students to lie down into a final Savasana, where they can rest deeply for a few minutes (with or without instrumental music), allowing their body and mind to integrate the benefits of the practice.

MINDFULNESS MOVEMENT CLASS: SELF-AWARENESS CLASS 1

This class complements the teachings on interoception, as it includes simplistic postures with a focus on sensory input. The Body Scan Exercise can be done before or after this class to foster interoception or embodied awareness.

Take a quick baseline of how you feel with three easy breaths.

PACING

As we move through our practice, be aware of the pace of your movements, as the speed of our actions affect our body and mind. For example, take a moment to reach your arm overhead, like you have a brilliant answer to the teacher's question, and then lower it back down. Now repeat that same movement, taking five or so slow breaths to reach as high as you can, then slowly lower it back down.

STUDENT REFLECTION

What did you notice about the two different ways you moved?

Most of the time, you'll be encouraged to move more slowly than usual to allow time and space for observation. Sometimes, however, moving fast is interesting too and can help relieve pent up emotion or stress from the body.

1. Child's pose with forehead on a block. This posture helps to calm our vagus nerve, a very important nerve in the body. It is the longest cranial nerve that runs throughout the body and influences all of the major functions such as digestion, our breathing, our heart rate and the way we deal with stress. People with healthy vagus nerve functioning are considered to have 'high vagal tone' and have the ability to quickly return to a balanced baseline. People who are more sensitive to stress may have 'low vagal tone', making it more difficult for them to regulate emotions and deal with life's challenges. Yoga and mindfulness help to balance the nervous system, giving it a chance to discharge stress. This posture is especially helpful for soothing the vagus nerve and we can enhance the calming effect even more by emphasizing our exhalations, letting them last longer than the inbreath. Quiet your thinking mind, release any thoughts, worries and concerns, as you connect to the still, grounding energy of mother earth.

2. Slowly rise to sitting and take a moment to quietly form an intention for your class that supports your wellbeing.

3. In Tadasana, begin your Sun Breath by inhaling arms overhead, exhaling hands together, gliding down your midline. Do these eight to ten more times to set a slow mindful pace and bring about an awareness of your inner most being. As you flow, draw your attention away from the outside world and into your center, the core of who you are.

4. Come to standing in Tadasana, cultivating the awareness of both stability and flexibility. Establish your awareness of your foundation through the feet, feeling grounded and strong. Your legs are like tree trunks, your knees are slightly bent, and your pelvis is neutral. Can you feel the stability at your center here? Your upper body is lightly lifting, as though being pulled upward by a puppet master above you. Can you feel the spaciousness in your spinal column and your torso? Take a few more breaths here, attempting to merge the qualities of stability with fluidity. Too much stability causes rigidity, while an excess of flexibility causes weakness. We need both elements to feel balanced in mind and body.

5. Take two to three Sun Breaths, mindful of sensation throughout your body and the flow of your breath.

6. Surya Namaskara very slowly
    a. First one, focus entirely on the inhalation and the exhalation. Can you notice how each aspect of the breath generates different energy and sensation?
    b. Next one, focus your complete awareness on your feet in Tadasana, facing forward, arches lifted while engaging your four-point stance or pada bandha.
    c. Next Namaskara, harness your attention on the kneecaps. In Tadasana visualize the top borders of your kneecaps moving back toward the thigh bones. Can you feel your thigh muscles engage, without locking out the knees? Keep this action throughout the sequence.
    d. Next one, focus completely on your mula bandha and Uddiyana bandha, while breathing smoothly. Can you maintain this gentle stabilizing engagement throughout the sequence?

7. Now draw your awareness to your shoulder blades, attempting to tuck the bottom ridge of your blades into your lower mid back. When you hug the shoulder blades onto your backside, what happens to your chest? What happens to your breathing? Maintain this action throughout your next namaskara.

8. Finally, let's view our bodies as the vehicle by which we experience the world around us. Without the physical body, we would not know the taste of ice cream, or the softness of a cozy blanket, or the smell of fresh mint, the beauty of a loved one's smile, or the melody of your favorite song. All of the senses are only experienced through the body, and only to the degree that we are present for them, as they arise in our lives Take a moment to land here, in the miraculous creation of your body. Right here, right now, one breath at a time...do a namaskara with this awareness.

9. Anchored in the awareness of your body, now let's expand our consciousness out beyond the self, to the space around us, near and far. Keep expanding your awareness until you see yourself within the context of the whole universe, about the size of the tip of a pen, and let yourself settle into this almost unfathomable perspective. The mind can become so consumed by the drama of our own lives that we forget to lift our gaze and meet other humans eye to eye, heart to heart. We miss out on the magic occurring right above our heads, as fluffy clouds float by and stars shimmer in the night sky. As you breathe here visualize yourself as one essential component within the great human story. Let yourself be comforted by this reality, you are a key player in the game of life. Also, allow yourself to be awe struck by the divine genius that created and continues to create this pulsing, living, breathing Universe. As we flow through our next namaskara, imagine your breath breathing all of life.

10. In Tadasana now, can you integrate all of these components so that we're aware of: our

breathing, our feet, our knee caps, our core bandhas, our shoulder blades, and our newly expanded awareness, which is the ultimate practice of yoga and mindfulness. Take a few deep breaths and soften any rigidity that was created from this exercise.

11. Come to sitting and find Staff pose/Dandasana
12. Seated forward bend/Paschimottanasana
13. Savasana- be still, soften your breath and allow relaxation to seep into your system.

MINDFULNESS MOVEMENT CLASS: SELF-AWARENESS CLASS 2

In a comfortable seated position, awaken your breathing body and form an intention for your time on your mat

1. Spinal undulations, inhaling as you arch, exhaling as you round the spine. Begin slowly and after a few minutes, increase your pace to build heat in the core, and then slow down your movements to eventually come to stillness.
2. Seated side stretch
3. Table to Cat/Cow
4. Standing Rag doll, hanging the head and arms, slowly curl up to Mountain Pose
5. Sun Salutations, recalling the focal points from last class: our breathing, our feet, our knee caps, our core bandhas, our shoulder blades, and our newly expanded awareness
6. Downward dog, inhale lift right leg into Extended Downward dog and step forward into lunge with back knee down, maintaining bandhas and neutral pelvis, sweep arms overhead for five breaths.
7. Release the left arm down and plant the left hand as you reach up with the right arm, lifting left knee if appropriate. Stay in this modified side angle twist for five breaths, bringing awareness to the feet, the knee caps, the bandhas and shoulder blade action.
8. Repeat the sequence on the other side.
9. Next vinyasa, inhale to Extended Downward dog, exhale and tuck the right knee into chest, inhale, sweep it out and back, rotating through the hip joint. Observe sensation in the hip and alignment of the upper body, evenly distributing body weight on both hands. Do this hip rotation three times, and on the final rotation, step forward into Warrior 1, arms wide overhead, breathing deeply into the awareness of points of the feet, the knee caps, the bandhas and shoulder blade action.
10. From Warrior 1, lift back heel and reach left arm across right thigh to revolved Side Angle, exploring arm variations. The goal is to rotate the spine to release tension and to create gentle compression of the abdominal organs. Remain for five to ten breaths, release out and do the same on the other side.
11. Balance postures: from Tadasana, shift your weight to the left foot and lift your right heel off the floor to introduce balancing on one foot to your nervous system. Breathe smoothly and return your awareness to the four points of the feet, the knee caps, the bandhas and shoulder blade action. Switch sides.
12. Stay with your breathing, as you slightly lift the right knee and interlock fingers around the upper shin. Hold for five or so breaths, then switch sides.
13. Dolphin plank: engaging the points of awareness at the feet, the knee caps, the bandhas and shoulder blade action. This posture really accents the action through the legs, core and shoulders. The challenge here is to remain strong while infusing this posture with ease and fluidity.
14. Relax on belly with hands under forehead and let the hips sway from side to side to release any tension or rigidity that may have snuck into your body.
15. Locust pose with arms alongside the torso or Flying Saucer with arms out from shoulders. Lift head, chest and legs off the ground to engage the backside and stretch the front body.
16. Reach both arms overhead in front of you, bringing palms together into Lahiri prostration

141

MINDFULNESS IN SCHOOLS MANUAL

and take time to give thanks for your life, for the guidance of a force greater than you and anything else you'd like to honor in this moment: a loyal friend, a loving family member, a dedicated teacher, or even your pet.

17. Child's pose/Balasana
18. Seated forward bend/Paschimottanasana
19. Supine Twist: breathing slowly now into the awareness of the points of the body that were our focus today, relaxing the feet and the knee caps. Release engagement of the bandhas by letting your belly relax and shoulders soften. Twist on both sides.
20. Rise to sitting for five finger mindfulness practice.

FIVE FINGER MINDFULNESS PRACTICE

Each finger represents an element in the natural world, and by touching each finger to the thumb, we bring our inner elements into balance. The fingertips are one of the most highly sensitized areas on the body. Therefore, hand and finger postures, called mudras open specific electromagnetic currents within the body and restore our health and balance.

1. Let's start our finger meditation by bringing your thumb and index finger together on each hand and rest your hands in your lap. Breathe slowly and deeply and notice the subtle sensations at the tips of your fingers and thumbs.
2. The thumb represents the fire element and the index finger represents the air we breathe and the joining of these two releases mental fog, sharpens our intellect and inspires happiness. Enjoy your breath here for a moment.
3. Thumbs now connect with middle finger, joining the fire element of the thumb with the element of space in the middle finger. Tension is contractive while space is expansive. Imagine your true essence expanding into the space element. Feel tension softening within your body as you rest your attention on the spaciousness of your breath.
4. Shift your thumbs now so they connect with your ring fingers, awakening a feeling of grounding and stability as you surrender to the force of gravity. Just simply watch your thoughts flow in and out of your mind as you acknowledge the rooting element of earth.
5. Let the thumbs make contact with the pinky fingers now, providing the body with the fluidity, adaptability and resilience of water. Focus here on the wave like action of your breath, on the ebb and flow of the in breath and the outbreath, as you imagine the subtle yet powerful quality of water flowing through you.
6. Finally, draw your hands together at heart center and feel your individual Self merging harmoniously with the elements of nature surrounding you. Feeling integrated, balanced and present, you can either close the class or if time allows, release back into Savasana.

MINDFULNESS MOVEMENT CLASS—SELF LOVE

Objectives

- Instill self-love
- Strengthen and harmonize the body/mind connection
- Calm the nervous system with long held postures
- Enhance breath awareness

SELF-LOVE QUIZ

This class is designed to encourage you to become more mindful of how you treat yourself on a daily basis. The more awareness we can shed on the treatment of ourselves, the more capable we are of making positive changes that support our health and happiness.

Start with this quiz It's designed to encourage you to become more mindful of how you engage with yourself on a daily basis. The more awareness we can bring to the way in which we treat ourselves, the more capable we are of making positive changes that foster self worth and self-love, resulting in greater health and happiness.

Studies show that people who are more compassionate and loving to themselves, experience more life success, more resilience, greater relationship fulfillment and deeper levels of inner peace. Mark your answers on a scale of 1 to 5.

1	2	3	4	5
Never	Rarely	Sometimes	Mostly	Always

Questions

Are you gentle with yourself throughout the day?	
Does your inner dialogue nurture your wellbeing?	
Do you do little acts of kindness for yourself?	
Do you let yourself receive a complement?	
Do you believe that being loving and gentle with yourself is healthy and natural?	
Do you respectfully listen to your own needs (instead of ignoring them and putting others needs before yours)?	
TOTAL SCORE	

Add up your score. The answers to these questions may reveal your level of self-love and the degree to which you care for yourself.

If you scored less than 11, you may be living in sparse, barren love conditions that require a big self-care renovation. Not to worry, you were born with love for yourself and therefore you still hold the memory of it inside. Life has just taken you off course a bit. Through this work, you will unlearn the lies you were told about yourself and discover the truth of who you really are, which is totally and immensely lovable.

If your score was between 12 and 20, you may be sometimes good to yourself, and sometimes rotten, so there are still improvements to be made in your generosity with yourself.

If your score was between 21 and 30, congratulations, you are living with a healthy amount of self-love, which tends to translate into good health physically, mentally, emotionally and spiritually.

YIN YOGA CLASS

1. Find Hero Pose with hands joined at heart center
   Opening affirmations and reflections;
   I realize that when I open my heart to Love, life surprises me with goodness.
   I know that I can only truly love another by finding peace within myself first.
2. Fan the heart fire by starting in Anjali mudra, and inhale hands apart, exhale palms together for five to ten cycles. Add affirmation: "Breathing in I honor my heart, breathing out I fill it with love."
3. Continue this movement as teacher reads the following dialogue:

   Now is the time for you to practice loving yourself. To be able to love another, you must be able to give love to yourself first Loving others means loving them exactly as they are and loving yourself means giving yourself the same gift Be with yourself here, as you are, with an attitude of love and acceptance. Appreciate the precious gift that you are. If you find this difficult to do, just pretend you are offering love to a loved one whom you adore, and just imagine what it would feel like to direct that love your way

   Our work on the mat tends to bring our brokenness to the surface, so that we can mend it with love. You are already perfect, you just need to reframe how you see yourself and you can do that by committing to self-love and changing how you talk to yourself. Throughout this class, notice your inner dialogue. When a harsh judgment or a comparison arises, observe it, but also question its truth. Eventually, as you fortify your commitment to self-love, you'll notice your inner dialogue becoming more compassionate, more generous and more loving.
4. Hero Pose: Interlock fingers with palms in your lap facing upward, inhale lift your hands up your mid-line turning palms open to gradually press overhead. Maintaining the interlock, exhale press palms out as you lower them back down. Take 5-10 breaths here.
5. Butterfly Pose (Cobbler's Pose): Come home to your body here and be mindful of how you're holding your body, how you're breathing your body. The body and its needs are so often overlooked, as we impress our minds goals on it. We push our body too far in exercise, or we don't give it enough activity, we under eat, we over eat, we consume foods and substances that intoxicate our body, and we all too often exhaust it through insufficient sleep. We spend too many wakeful hours immersed in distractions such as work, socialization and entertainment. We alienate our bodies from our day to day life experience, we disassociate from parts of the body that hold unfavorable memories, and we numb sensations and override messages with prescription drugs, sugar, caffeine or alcohol so we don't have to listen to its requests. Our society today profits on self-hatred and body dissatisfaction, and so we're encouraged to criticize and condemn our bodies.

   We can be so punishing to our bodies, not because we don't care, but because we don't know how to love and accept our bodies, as they are. We don't give ourselves permission to celebrate our bodies because we're told to strive for unrealistic standards of perfection. All of this hatred and rejection of the body has a powerful energetic effect, dis-eased thinking leads to dis-eased cells.

   It is possible to turn the wheel on this momentum of body hatred and the first step is to consider the practice of being grateful for the body you have been given, not the body you could have if you worked a few more hours a week, not the body you might have if you got this or that cosmetic surgery done, but your body right here, right now.

Your body is brilliant, it is one of the most genius machines on the planet, able to instantaneously attack incoming viruses and bacteria, digest food, secrete the right hormone in just the right amount in any given moment, all at the same time! With the 10 million diseases we could contract, it's a miracle that our bodies operate as well as they do!

6. Sphinx Pose: Breathe into the belly, into the heart and practice self-acceptance, self-compassion and self-love.

   Consider the possibility that there is nothing you need to change about your body in order to love it…that you could love and accept your body just as it is, in all its uniqueness, right now.

7. Child's Pose: As we peel away the physical layers of tension, we discover who we really are and what we're truly made of. Going deeper in a pose doesn't mean that we max out our stretch, it means that we deepen our experience of love and deepen our understanding of ourselves.

8. Dragon Pose: Dialogue for first side: nothing worthwhile has ever come out of criticism, judgment and scrutiny. We don't awaken our inner light through force or tough love, in fact, addictive and obsessive behaviour seems to flourish when these are present. As yogis, we fertilize the soil of our body with compassion, tenderness and love, acceptance for ourselves as we are right now.

   Dialogue for second side: if you're longing to feel okay, just as you are, you are in the right place, for this comfort can be found within. This journey is not about adding anything at all, but more about letting go, letting go of negativity and all that doesn't serve you. By clearing away the falsities, what remains is you in all your brilliance. Our work then is not to change or become someone else, but rather to simply let ourselves be exactly who we are.

   Twisted dragon
   I can only truly connect with another
   By becoming present to myself.
   I can only truly love another
   By filling my own heart with love.
   When I open my heart to Love
   I am filled with delight and peace.

9. Swan Pose (Pigeon Pose): With crossed wings to open the back door of the heart. Let go of the pain from the past so you can enjoy the love that is here for you today.

10. Caterpillar (Seated Forward Bend): Today you are invited to say goodbye to feeling bad about your body and your appearance Today is your opportunity to stop colluding with a culture that profits on your pain by convincing you to feel inadequate. It's time to say goodbye to your inner critic, the one who keeps you striving and never lets you just be in peace. Your inner critic has meant well, but the true path to love is through radical self-acceptance. It's radical because it's not the norm, we twist self-acceptance into a concept that implies apathy or laziness.

   But to be radically self-accepting, is to be gentle with yourself, to be forgiving with yourself, to be generous with yourself and to love and accept yourself for who you are right now.

   The next time you see your reflection in the mirror, listen for the story line you tell yourself: that you're too fat or too rolly, too boring or too average, too old, or too saggy. And just listen to the story, like standing at the edge of a pool, and choosing to look at the water without jumping in.

The next time you see yourself in a mirror, just simply see your face, your body, your temple. When you stop yourself from jumping into the pool of self-criticism, what you start to see then is the real you, the you that shines with beauty, and lightness and uniqueness. And that is the first step toward healing your relationship with your body and transforming your experience of the world.

11. Pentacle (Corpse Pose): Let's take a pledge together to be kinder to ourselves. As we do that, just imagine the people in our lives who will also be affected by this paradigm shift.

Your family, your children, your friends, your colleagues, your students will all benefit from this new sense of being at peace within yourself, and you will naturally help to elevate their relationship to their body. By healing our relationship with our body, we contribute to spreading peace throughout the world.

12. Closing Affirmation

I am worthy of the same love I give to others.

I welcome goodness and love into my life.

I choose to feel good about who I am.

MINDFULNESS MOVEMENT CLASS – ANXIETY CALMING CLASS

This class complements the section on anxiety and stress.

Objectives

- Liberate trapped energy stuck in upper body
- Soothe the nervous system with slow, repetitive movements
- Enhance body awareness
- Relax over-all tension patterns

Anxiety is a mental health concern that is growing in our young people today for many reasons, a few being the uncensored exposure to negative and adult news, technology overload, the unreasonable standard of perfection that is impressed upon them and a lack of spiritual/social support. Anxiety is described as an overall feeling of worry, tension and concern stemming from a feeling of lack of control. Often the source of anxiety seems unclear and hard to pinpoint because it can linger for long periods of time.

As a group: How would you describe anxiety?

In partners:

- What are some anxiety triggers that you face in an average day? Which ones are real and which ones are contrived by your imagination?
- When anxiety arises, what sensations do you experience in your body and mind?
- How do you currently manage anxiety? Is it helpful? Is it skillful?

According to Lisa M. Schab, in the Anxiety workbook for teens, anxiety is dependent on four factors: genetics, brain chemistry, life experiences and personality.

We can't control the first three factors, but we can work on our personality. Through mindfulness, we learn to train our mind and focus our thoughts, which help to cultivate a peaceful state within the body. By practicing these skills before an anxiety causing event, we prepare ourselves, just as an athlete would prepare for a competition. Therefore, when a trigger arises, we can draw on our training and react in a more skillful way.

According to Ayurveda, anxiety is a Vata condition often caused from being over-scheduled, chronically stressed and having an over-active mind. We are not designed to spend as much time in our heads as we do today and as a result, we are neglecting our bodies and our breath We need to shift our energy from the obsessive tendency of the mind and anchor our attention in our body so we can better meet its needs and re-establish balance This class is designed to release held tension that traps our energy in the head and draw it down into the lower reaches of the body.

Starting with breath awareness, take a moment to imagine if you were held under water for any period of time? You'd panic, right? That's how so many of us are living our lives as we unconsciously hold our breath. Holding our breath to deal with life's challenges is dangerously unhealthy, putting tremendous pressure on the heart and adversely affecting other organs. Alas there are more effective ways of dealing with stress, and it all starts with mindful awareness of the breath and how we hold our bodies.

1. Start by lying on your belly, practicing deep breathing, with hands under forehead. Let your belly completely relax into your mat, letting go of tension in your abdomen, letting go of the effort to be something you're not, like trying to be skinnier, or smarter than you really are, let it go and relax. This is time for you to give yourself permission to just be you. Take five minutes here noticing your front body in contact with the earth and let yourself melt downward. Become aware of your back body now, using your five senses and your sixth sense of intuitive knowing to become totally aware of how you feel in this moment. Keep breathing smoothly, and if any discomfort, physical or emotional, arises, try exhaling fluidly and deeply and let it pass through you.

2. Roll onto your back and move into single leg apanasana/knee to chest into supine twist. Invite the heart to expand breath by breath, holding each pose for five or so breaths and switch sides.

3. Press up to hero pose and begin full yogic breathing, with an even measure of the inbreath and outbreath, adding the Heart/Gut gesture by placing one hand on heart and one hand on lower abdomen to palpate your breathing.

4. Shoulder shrugs and neck stretches

5. Table to cat/cow

6. Table, side plank either with top foot to floor or both legs straight, to wild thing with top foot behind top arm arching overhead.

7. Downward dog to Mountain Pose/Tadasana

8. Shake it out: bouncing to shake out hands, legs and head, gently. Add vocalization on the exhalation, sigh loudly, blubber the lips and encourage laughter.

9. Lifting up the sky: interlock fingers and reach palms overhead, exhale sweep arms out and down, five times. Next five breaths, add a lift in the heels, rising up on balls of feet as you inhale and exhale lower the arms and rest on your feet again Do these movements slowly, honing your awareness of balance and breath.

10. Arm swinging, forward and back to move energy.

11. Standing side stretch/half-moon/banana

12. Back to Mountain Pose, notice if you have any more freedom to stand tall and breathe deeply, this is good!

13. Wide legged squat with twist

14. Utkatasana twists to standing forward bend/Uttanasana

15. Gather and ground your energy: reach arms out and up above the head with palms down, fingers touching, and exhale lower the hands down front body as though pressing a beach ball down under water. Do this 3x and rest hands on lower belly. Observe where your energy is focused now. Are you feeling more grounded and in your body?

16. Tree pose, being cautious of keeping your energy rooted as you extend the arms overhead.

17. Cobra to child's vinyasa, 5-10x

18. Child's pose with head on block or hands to soothe the vagus nerve at forehead, this same pose can be done at their desks if they notice a need to calm down arises.

19. Apanasana: Squeeze your nose into your knees and contract every muscle in your body, tight, tight, tight, imagining all of your anxiety, and nervousness curling into a ball at your core and then exhale and let it go as you unravel your body. As you release back into an outstretched position, let the ball roll out of you, off your mat, and out of the room.

20. Savasana: calming the body for relaxation or sleep is not something you can make happen, there's nothing you can 'do' about it. It's more about letting go and allowing calm to enter your system.

21. Closing: Hands at heart center, close your eyes and slow your breathing. Remind yourself that you are enough and all is well.

MINDFULNESS MOVEMENT CHAIR CLASS FOR EMOTIONAL REGULATION

This chair class can be done in its entirety or one posture at a time, as needed. Chair postures are a wonderful way of incorporating movement into the classroom, while teaching students the importance of taking energy breaks throughout the day.

The limbic system is the portion of the fore brain that is known as the center of our emotions. To function optimally, the structures within the limbic system require an even flow of energy throughout our body's systems. When stressors disturb our lives, tension blocks energy flow as well as blood circulation, like a kink in a hose. When energy flow is obstructed, we can feel mentally foggy, emotionally imbalanced and physically off center. Your emotions are natural by products to life's varied experiences, and they reflect our inner reality moment to moment.

We've all experienced extreme emotion at one time or another in our lives. Do you remember how you felt after the intense emotion subsided? An emotional outburst of any kind, whether its sadness or excitement, can cause imbalance in our system, leaving us feeling fatigued and drained. When we over-indulge our emotions, we pour fuel on our emotional flames, stimulating the emotional center of the brain and training it to react just as strongly the next time.

Alternatively, if we have been conditioned to 'Stop crying' when disturbing life experiences strike, we may have trained ourselves to contract and numb out in order to deal with emotional upheaval. When we do this, our body adapts by tensing muscles, trapping emotional patterns and trauma in our cellular make up. Just as emotions shape our face, with worry lines and smile creases, our emotions can deeply affect our internal organs too.

The following gentle movement sequence is designed to release tension within the body through easy and accessible chair poses. When muscles relax, energy can flow and the mind and emotions can return to their natural state of balance.

EMOTIONAL ENERGY SCAN, EITHER SEATED OR IN SAVASANA

The body tends to retain emotional energy in the hips, belly, heart, throat and jaw. Let's start the process by drawing your attention to your hips and pelvis. Do you notice any emotional energy hiding out there? When you find something, like discomfort or sensation, just keep exhaling to release it.

What about your belly? We tend to carry anxiety and nervousness here. Respond to your discoveries with deep, slow breathing and a non-judgmental attitude.

When suppressed, we often hide our emotions in the deep layers of the heart. Rest a hand on your heart and patiently watch to see what surfaces. Keep breathing, slowly, peacefully as you gently knock on the door of your emotions. They have been so comfortable lying dormant within this treasure chest, so don't poke or pry it open, just knock and gently dust it off.

Rise up to the region of your throat and jaw, where we communicate with the world around us. How effectively do you verbalize your truth? Are you open to hearing it from others? Too often we bite our tongue, keeping our true reality caged inside so we don't offend anyone. Maybe we don't believe we are deserving of a better situation. Can you affirm to yourself that you are safe to soften and relax this area? Imagine tension just evaporating with each exhalation.

Notice your third eye, do you hold tension behind the eyes? This is the area where we tend to create stories about life and people, so don't intellectualize this experience, just observe the nature of mind and encourage stillness.

Our intention is to free ourselves of emotional constriction and the resulting muscular tension. We don't need to push or force it out, but rather invite its release.

Emotions can be elusive; they're not like a dog that comes running when we call. We may need to do some mining to uncover and release them. You can ask yourself as we go along, is this the right time to let this go? Do I deserve happiness? Transformation will occur when you're ready, so keep moving toward it.

1. Start with the individual practice of full yogic breathing and incorporate circular breathing, becoming aware of holding patterns and tension that may be blocking the smooth flow of the breath.

2. Find a partner and sit back to back. Become present the rhythm of your own breathing, then become aware of your partners breathing and notice if your breathing starts to synchronize.

3. Rise to standing and identify a partner A and a partner B.

   Part 1: partner A practices full yogic breathing while partner B stands behind and rests hands on the lower back, encouraging partner A to fill the belly with breath and partner B's hands with each inbreath.

   Part 2: partner A practices full yogic breathing, filling their belly and adding expansion of the ribs while partner B stands behind and places hands on partner A's ribs. Partner A practices breathing into their hands in the inbreath and moves ribs away from their hands on the outbreath.

   Part 3: partner A breathes into upper lungs while partner B stands beside partner A and rests a finger on partner A's sternum and the other hand on their upper back/nape of the neck. Partner A attempts to fill their lungs to press into their partners hands and move away from their contact on the outbreath.

   Discuss with your partner what you noticed about your breathing with this support. Switch roles.

4. In a chair, come to the front edge of your seat so your spine can lengthen without a back rest. Find your natural breath here, relax your shoulders away from your ears and form a personal intention for your time of mindful movement.

5. Shoulder shrugs 3x

6. Neck stretches

7. Playfully explore "face yoga" by reciting together the vowels: A, E, I, O, U, pronounce each vowel in the most exaggerated fashion to loosen the jaw, stretch the muscles in the face and hopefully have a good laugh.

8. Cat/Cow with hands on your thighs to awaken the spine.

9. Seated Twist—turning to the side of your chair, twist backwards with both hands on the backrest. Switch sides.

10. Seated forward bend—inhale reach arms overhead, exhale fold over your bent legs and allow your head to hang. Inhale rise back up with arms reaching tall, exhale arms down, back to an upright seated position.

11. Namaskara/salutation using the chair:

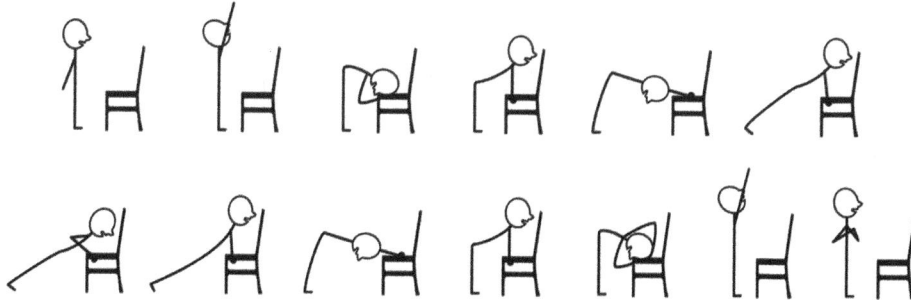

a) Standing forward bend with hands clasping opposite elbows, resting elbows on backrest or seat of chair, calming the monkey mind with this gentle inversion.

b) Curl up, vertebra by vertebra to mountain pose

c) Modified upward dog with both hands on the seat of the chair, drawing hips forward and arching spine to gaze upward. Arms and legs are straight, weightbearing on the toes.

d) Seated Warrior 1 and lunge

e) Seated Warrior 2 and Side Angle

f) Core lift—sit on the edge of your chair and press your hands into the sides of your seat to lift your hips up. Hold for 5 breaths, lower and repeat.

g) Balasana/child's pose –come in close to your desk, make a pillow with your hands and rest your forehead on your hands.

h) Seated Savasana—sitting back so your spine is supported, close your eyes and exhale with Fall Out breaths to calm your system. Rest here for a few moments before re-entering classroom activity.

Art Therapy and Mindful Movement Class 1

by Talia Carin, Art therapist (AT), Canadian Certified Counsellor (CCC), Naturotherapist (ND) and Registered Yoga Teacher, https://www.montrealtherapy.com/?s=talia+carin

Class Theme

Visualizing the breath

Props/Materials

Blocks, straps, markers, chalk, or coloured pencils, large roll of paper, body outline templates (2 per student). See the end of this lesson for a handout.

Invite each individual to select 2 drawing materials (2 pencils or 2 markers, etc.) and to cut a piece of paper large enough for each of them to sit in the middle of it and be able to extend their arms in all directions without leaving the page.

Introduce the concept of a kinesphere—created by Rudolf Laban. Defined as "the sphere around the body whose periphery can be reached by easily extended limbs without stepping away from that place which is the point of support when standing on one foot". This spherical space around our body shifts as soon as we shift our weight. It is also the first area of movement exploration before going into space in general.

Emphasize that this is an exploration, there is no right or wrong way to do it. Start by sitting comfortably, with a drawing tool of the same colour in each hand and with the hands extended in front of you. Slowly inhale, reaching the arms back at the same pace of the breath. When you get to the end of your breath, pause for a second and then begin to exhale slowly while drawing the hands back together in front of you. Take a moment to look at the shape you have drawn. This is the visual expression of your breathing. Now continue to do this for 10 breaths. See if you can extend the breath and the movement to be wider, reaching further back, or further out to the side. See how it feels to slow it down, or to speed it up.

Centering with Intention

> Yoga is the artwork of awareness being painted on the canvas of the body, mind and soul. ~ Dr.Amit Ray. Indian author and spiritual teacher.

Invite people to talk about what this means to them, how they interpret it. Does the visual of painting awareness onto aspects of the self appeal to them?

Start in Savasana with a guided body scan, inviting attention to where they might feel buzzing, tension, tingling, pressure, energy, etc. In your mind's eye, focus on one area of heightened sensation. Does it look or feel different from the rest of your body? Does it seem light or dark? Is there a specific colour to it? Is there increased energy here, or a blockage of energy? Does it have a shape? Search for another area in your body that has a lot of sensation.

How might you describe this feeling? Does it have a special color, shape, or energy that is unique to this area?

Note: as they rest in reflection, pass out the body template handouts (drawing material will already be out). Once the scan is finished, invite them to gently open their eyes and rise to sitting. They can now fill in the first body template based on whatever shape, texture or colour they may have experienced during the guided body scan. No facial features, details, etc. Mention that they may not have visualized anything and that's totally ok.

1. Namaskara A
2. Namaskara B: As the class does this, invite them to think about the sensations generated throughout the body, noticing the intensity, colour, shape, or texture of the energy.
3. Mountain-Tadasana
4. Vinyasa 1
5. Low lunge-Anjaneyasana to Warrior 1
6. Repeat sequence on left
7. Lower yourself to the mat or vinyasa down.
8. Vinyasa 2
9. Warrior 2 to Triangle Pose to Half Moon/Ardha Chandrasana
10. Repeat sequence on left
11. Lower yourself to the mat or vinyasa down.
12. Locust Pose/Salabhasana
13. Bow Pose/Dhanurasana
14. Table to Cat/Cow pose
15. Downward dog/Adho Mukha Svanasana
16. Jump through to seated or step through.
17. Boat/Navasana to lying on the back.
18. Closing
19. Happy baby
20. Savasana (sleeping sloth/Corpse pose)
21. Think about any sensations you may be feeling in the body or in the mind.
22. Come out gently and complete a second body map. It may be the same, it may be different.

Invite students to share about the process if they feel comfortable doing so.

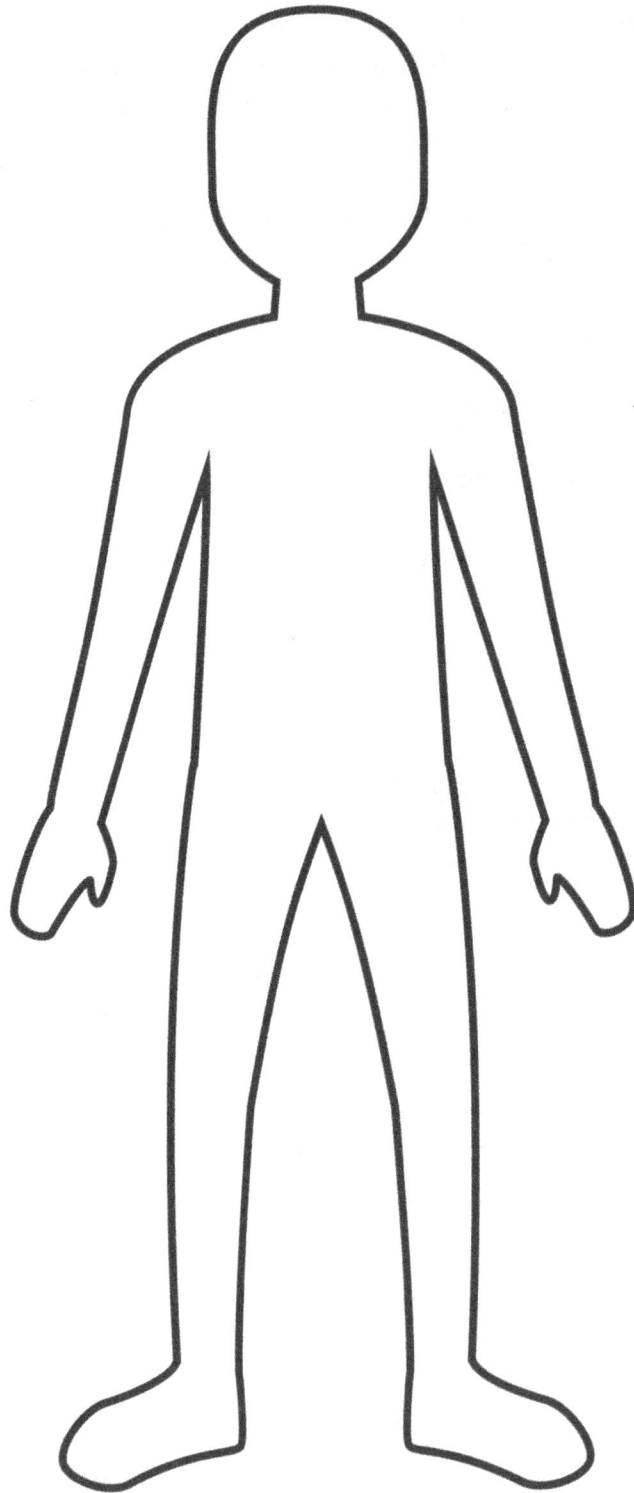

ART THERAPY AND MINDFUL MOVEMENT CLASS 2

by Talia Carin, Art therapist (AT), Canadian Certified Counsellor (CCC), Naturotherapist (ND) and Registered Yoga Teacher

CLASS THEME

Cultivating the observing self/non-judgment

PROPS/MATERIALS

Natural objects (rocks, shells, bark, etc.), blank paper and writing implement, blocks, straps.

This could be used as a warm up, to generate heat in the body, or could be a good way to introduce people to focusing on their breath. It would be great for people who are visual and kinesthetic learners, or who have a more concrete way of thinking. You could really play with it, inviting people to change colours depending on how fast they want to do the breathing, or have each person in group select a different colour so that in the end you have a beautiful visual representation of different energies and breaths in the room.

It would also be a great way to explore the concept of personal space and shared space in a classroom.

Feel free to suggest that the students overlap into each other's bubbles a bit to introduce the concept of personal and shared space. They can paint their own kinesphere however they wish and then work together to decide how to negotiate the shared space.

OBJECTIVE

Students will explore the theme of non-judgment first with a neutral object and then with themselves.

Introduction of theme: Invite group or individual to select an object from those provided; whatever stands out or appeals to them at this moment. Go onto your mat, place the object in your hands and close your eyes. Move the object around in your hands and notice all you can about it. As you begin to formulate a description of the object you've chosen, leave out words like "beautiful, perfect, nice or ugly", as these are considered value judgments. No value judgments, simply descriptive adjectives, such as; heavy, smooth, light, rough, cold, warm. Notice anything that arises for you during this process. Now repeat this process with your eyes open. Record the many non-value characteristics you came up with on the piece of paper provided.

Now reflect, has this exercise changed how you feel about your object at all?

In today's practice, we're going to retain this nonjudgmental attitude and apply it to ourselves.

1. Seated-neck stretches
2. Seated side bend.

3. Namaskara A
4. Namaskara B: As students go through their Namaskaras, invite them to think about non-valued descriptors for their bodies in different postures.
5. Forward fold/Padangusthasana
6. High lunge/Anjaneyasana
7. Revolved Side Angle/Parivrtti Parsvakonasana
8. Tree/Vrksasana
9. Plankasana to Side Plank/Vashistasana
10. Vinyasa back to standing.
11. Repeat on left side.
12. Camel Pose/Ustrasana
13. Child's Pose/Balasana
14. Seated Forward bend/Paschimottanasana
15. Head to knee forward bend/Janu Sirsasana
16. Supine Twist
17. Savasana
18. Closing quote: Don't try to be anything. Do not make yourself into anything. Do not be a meditator. Do not be enlightened. When you sit, let it be. When you walk, let it be. Grasp at nothing. Resist Nothing."-Ajahn Chah (Thai Buddhist monk)

Invite participants to reflect on what they observed from doing this practice. They can write down any non-valued descriptors that they chose to describe their own body, or sensations as they practiced.

Was it easy to come up with the words? Was it difficult to do so while practicing? Was it hard to find non-valued descriptors for their body? How was it in comparison to choosing words for the natural, unbiased object?

MINDFULNESS MOVEMENT CLASS—MINDFUL WALKING PRACTICE

LOCATION

On a smooth terrain, preferably in a quiet area where you won't be expected to engage socially with others.

EQUIPMENT

Good footwear such as walking sneakers as there is a balance component to this type of slow movements.

TIMER

It is recommended to give yourself a specific start and finish so you can be fully present without concern about the time frame.

The first time I did a walking meditation it felt as though I was racing the tour de France and had just blown a tire…slow was so unfamiliar to me, not only to my mind that had become accustomed to racing but to my body as well, which I had trained for the first 20 years of my life as an elite athlete to operate at full throttle Over the agonizing period of an hour, going nowhere slowly, a very interesting thing happened. My initial frustration and impatience evolved into a manifesto of new sensations and discoveries about myself. You too may find this practice immensely challenging, because life in our western world is so over-scheduled that we have to go at top speed to accomplish it all.

Whether we're students rushing to complete assignments on time, parents speeding through the grocery isles or professionals focused on work efficiency, our bodies are conditioned for speed. In this society, hustle equals success whereas slow means unproductive, (ever notice we use the term 'slow' to refer to a person who is mentally delayed?).

But let's talk a bit about the stress crisis we're currently facing. Stress is the number one killer today in developing countries, the culprit behind cardiovascular disease, cancer, diabetes, obesity, anxiety disorders and the list goes on. When we really stop, or at least slow down and think about it, we can see just how devastating this pace is for our bodies, our minds and our spirits.

The body needs oxygen that can only be gleaned through deep, full breathing, it's not a 'nice to have', it's a requirement for life! The mind operates optimally by focusing on one thing at a time, just one thing. Multi-tasking doesn't make us more productive--the stress of it actually dulls our intellect and our memory.

The spiritual part of us requires leisure time with which to reflect, dream and just BE. Without this time, we become robotic in our lives, void of creativity and passion. So while this exercise may challenge every cell of your being and every belief you hold about how one should move in the world, take heart and know that you are doing a very healthy, natural thing for yourself. Moving slowly not only counters the devastating effects of stress, it will prolong your life and its quality. So many of us are living at such a speed that we have very superficial memories of daily life experiences. You will likely find as you become more mindful and present to your life that the moments you might have once categorized as mundane are now logged in as lasting memories.

What's so powerful about this type of mindfulness practice is how it involves the body. Yes we involve the body when we do our mindful movement practice, but walking is a function of our everyday lives. With each step, we have the opportunity to observe ourselves doing one of the most common movements done repeatedly each day, and largely unconsciously. Nothing in life can be changed until we become aware of it first.

As you walk, you can turn your awareness to your breathing. Over time, you'll likely notice how shallow or irregular your breathing is and how it gradually syncopates with the rhythm of your gate.

As you mindfully walk, you can observe how you're holding your body. This is a wonderful opportunity to correct habitual posture issues such as

- Forward head thrust where the head rests in front of your spine
- Slouching or rounded shoulders, causing your chest muscles tighten and shorten and the back muscles to lengthen and weaken
- Posterior tilt of the pelvis, which over stretches the spinal muscles and shortens the abdominal muscles, often caused from tight hamstrings
- Anterior tilt of the pelvis, which compresses the lumbar spine and weakens core stability
- Lateral imbalances that cause us to live more dominantly on one side than the other Technique:
- Arm variations: Clasp hands behind your back or interlock fingers in front of you, or simply let your arms hang freely to your sides.

Begin by standing tall and take a few deep, cleansing breaths to set the tone for your walk. You may notice yourself becoming so consumed in technique that you forget to breathe, which is a perfect time to remind yourself that the practice involves harmonizing your breath with your body movements.

To enhance the feeling tone of peace and pleasure that eventually comes from this practice, you may wish to maintain a slight grin on your face.

After a few centering breaths in Mountain Pose, you can gently bend your knees and slowly lift one foot off the ground so that your full weight transfers to the stabilizing leg. Slowly step forward and plant your foot in a heel to toe fashion. As you plant your heel and roll onto the ball of the foot, notice the sensations that this weight bearing action elicits along the foot bed. As your front foot plants, bend your front knee to absorb the weight and lift your back foot off the ground. Mindfully step your back foot forward and gently tap the toes beside your front foot. This tapping action mid stride is called pointing. After you point with the lifted leg, continue to step it forward and plant. Continue this cycle for as long as you have.

Observe the nature of your inner dialogue without impulsively acting on it. For example, you may notice habitual self-talk that sounds like "I have to hurry to get from point A to B in order to get it all done, or to get ahead, or to be loved and accepted." For all intents and purposes here, walking in this moment is the point, there is no point B, no finish line, you're simply walking for the sake of walking. Chances are you'll only walk about 40-50 feet in an hour-long practice anyway. But there is a physical benefit you may notice; slowly walking changes it from an aerobic workout to a strength building workout, requiring your leg muscles to contract isometrically to maintain balance.

As you walk, become curious about the different phases of walking and how you execute them. Do you notice that a certain part of your gate is faster and more unconscious than others? You may find it easier to be mindful during the planting phase when there's heightened sensation and feedback from the earth, while the transition phase might be more rushed as you pull your back foot into view for your senses to experience it.

I personally found that my transition was speedy, like I was trying to cheat where I could, and then slow on the heel to foot roll.

What other details do you notice about your walking experience? How are your socks fitting, are there any creases? Do you feel any hot spots on your feet as you walk?

What sounds do you notice? If you're outside, observe the lyrical sounds of nature with birds singing and squirrels chatting. If you do this practice first thing in the morning you can observe the many changes in color shades as the sun rises into the sky.

Instead of feeling self-conscious about neighbors catching you creeping robotically down the side walk, you can rest assured that your practice of moving slowly will affect their nervous systems as well, perhaps encouraging them to be more mindful about the pace in which they live.

Over time, you may notice yourself wanting to do the rest of your day at that pace, with deep, mindful breaths, a slow, rhythmic heart rate and a calm, focused mind.

PILLAR 3
INTRODUCTION TO COGNITIVE THERAPY

WHAT IS COGNITIVE THERAPY?

Cognitive therapy is a form of psychotherapy based on the concept that the way we think about things affects how we feel emotionally. It focuses on present time thinking and action. It emphasizes the importance of being in the here and now rather than focusing on past experiences. Cognitive Therapy, CT for short, is about problem solving, orienting the individual toward solutions to the challenges he/she is facing. It aims to help people in the ways they think (the cognitive component) and in the ways they act (the behavior component). The underlying assumption is that our thinking processes play an important role in the development and continuation of anxiety, depression, low self-esteem, negative self-image, substance abuse and dependence, aggression, relationship difficulties, etc.

WHY IS COGNITIVE THERAPY EFFECTIVE IN SCHOOLS?

The current school system is failing many students. They are coming to school and facing conflict with teachers, administrators and authorities on a daily basis with each trying to have his/her needs met, sometimes at the expense of others Because Cognitive Therapy is oriented toward problem solving, developing self-awareness, and changing negative thinking and behavior, it is the perfect adjunct to mindfulness training for fostering positive behaviors and a sense of wellbeing among student populations.

Additionally, the relationships among students, teachers and administrators have greater potential to develop into a more peaceful, happier, productive learning environment when all are practicing cognitive therapeutic and mindfulness techniques. Through these teachings we are able to better regulate our emotional landscape and realize that the outside world does not have absolute power to influence our state of being Cognitive therapy is more effective in a school setting, as you are dealing with the issue at hand, whereas psychotherapy is a longer process that can dive into long standing issues, such as traumatic stress.

William Glasser, the well-known CT practitioner and author, noted that although humans have developed and advanced their technological knowledge to include space travel, the internet, etc and made some improvements to society regarding social justice issues, 'we are no more able to get along with each other than we were before.' Conflicts everywhere seem to be escalating: the environment is in crisis, countries are still at war and domestic violence is a persistent problem.

I, Blair, work in schools and have yet to hear a teacher say things are better now than when he or she started teaching. Actually, I hear more of the opposite – that children's plights are more stressful than ever before. As a result, stress levels among teachers are at an all-time high.

Where do most of the problems originate? Most problems in life come right down to the relationships we have with others and the relationship we have with ourselves. If we look at how and why we experience conflict in our lives, we find that conflicts are relationship dependent, with each person striving to satisfy basic needs in a world of individuals who, for the most part, are unaware of the needs of those around them.

While relationships are central to many of our problems, they are often the most effective solution as well. Using a cognitive therapy inspired approach, the worksheets in this manual will provide teachers and students with solution-oriented tools to gain greater understanding of how they relate to others and how, through self-knowledge, to resolve and avoid conflicts.

Through this work, students learn to develop their internal self-control become more self-directed, confident, and take personal responsibility for the choices they make. This will empower them to develop healthier relationships, and to set realistic, achievable goals for a happier, more rewarding life. This is the art of mindfulness in action.

WHAT MAKES US "ACT"?

Each day teachers have conflicts with students. Students, in turn, have conflicts with each other, siblings, parents, etc. We frequently blame others for our moods, for making us feel the way we feel, but is that really fair or even accurate?

Let's look at what happens, for example, when a telephone rings. We might look at the call display and, rather than simply respond to the stimulus of the ringing phone by automatically answering it, decide whether we want to answer it or not at that particular moment in time. We might recognize a telemarketer number, a colleague we have no desire to speak to, or it may be a person we'd really like to connect with at that moment.

The life choices we make are based on complex internally-generated cognitive processes that can be influenced by our emotional state and life experiences. As students develop self-awareness and personal agency {do people know what this is?}, they realize that their lives as burgeoning adults are a compilation of choices that they make each and every day. While children are at the mercy of the situations they were born into, adults have the autonomy to choose. Sadly, many people live out their lives without this awareness, blaming others for their limitations and challenges.

The Cognitive Therapy approach is based on the theory that we are internally motivated to respond to the world around us and make choices based on our own intrinsic needs and desires. The CT inspired worksheets with this manual offer guidance for making choices and decisions that will enhance a person's life by helping them to make long-lasting, meaningful changes.

CT maintains that while there are many influences that affect our sense of agency {again should we use this term?} and personal power, (such as family conditioning, racial background and economic status to name a few) we are ultimately in the driver's seat, responsible for how we feel, act and react. Therefore, we can choose to make necessary adjustments in our thinking and our behavior to improve a situation at any time. Mindfulness training supports this approach by offering individuals simple methods to help them reflect on their behavior, consider the values and needs of others and incorporate heightened awareness into their day-to-day activities.

OUR BASIC NEEDS - POWERFUL FORCES THAT DRIVE US

Each day we are intrinsically motivated to satisfy our many needs. Each of our actions is carried out to satisfy one of these basic needs. Once we understand that we are driven by these needs, we can use this awareness to live a more satisfying and productive life.

MASLOW'S HIERARCHY OF NEEDS FOR THE CLASSROOM - MESSAGE FROM BLAIR

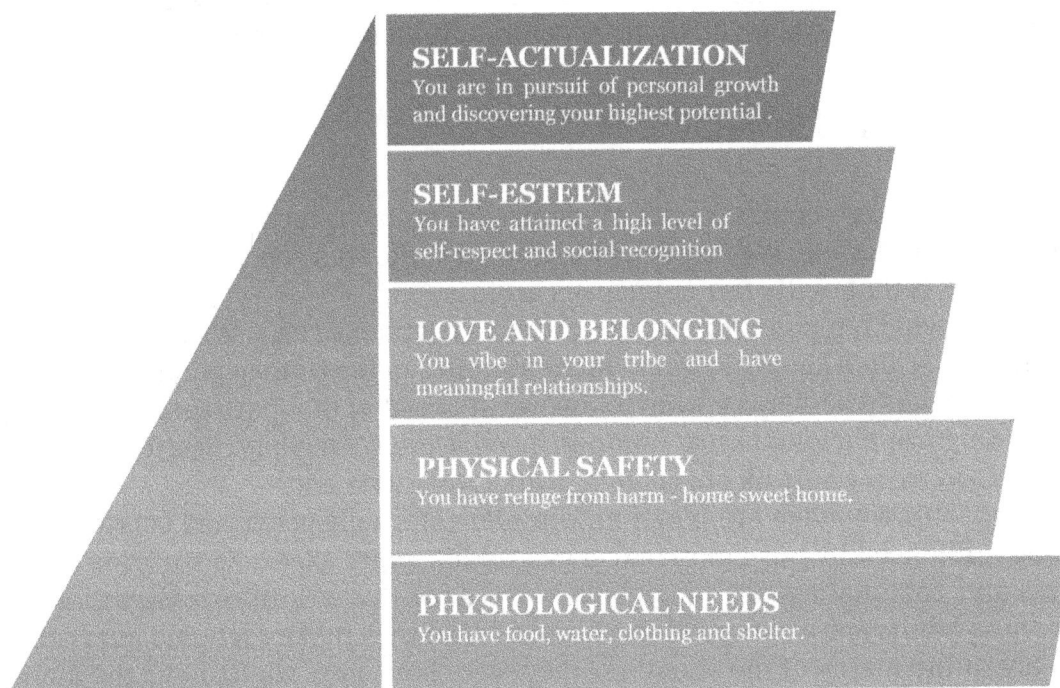

SELF-ACTUALIZATION
You are in pursuit of personal growth and discovering your highest potential.

SELF-ESTEEM
You have attained a high level of self-respect and social recognition

LOVE AND BELONGING
You vibe in your tribe and have meaningful relationships.

PHYSICAL SAFETY
You have refuge from harm - home sweet home.

PHYSIOLOGICAL NEEDS
You have food, water, clothing and shelter.

One of my best class management techniques was to begin each school year with the teachings of Maslow's hierarchy of needs. Most marketers use this structure to entice young and old to purchase products that claim to miraculously feed the void inside. I used it to help empower young minds to understand how our needs are the driving motivation behind everything we do. You can use the following lesson plan to help your class understand what motivates them during a typical day at school and what needs they are trying to satisfy when one student creates a disturbance in class while another quietly attempts to disappear.

With the diagram below, introduce Abraham Maslow, an American psychologist passionate about mental health and human potential, who proposed that humans have a hierarchy of needs which he presented in a five-tiered structure. As a first-generation Jewish boy in New York, Maslow was fiercely bullied which some say informed his thesis of human needs that he presented in a pyramid.

Starting at the bottom with physiological needs, Maslow claimed these are the basic requirements for survival, such as food, water, clothing and shelter.

Once this need is met, we move onto the need for physical safety, or refuge from harm.

When our physical safety need is fulfilled, we move onto the need to feel loved and belong to a group or tribe of some kind.

Moving up, we arrive at self-esteem, where we experience a feeling of regard for ourselves and we trust that others do as well.

The top of the pyramid is self-actualization, where we reach our highest human potential and attain deep understanding of the meaning of life.

After presenting the pyramid, you once again return to the bottom, inquiring with the students "When would someone's basic need for food, clothing and shelter be compromised?" Lead them to the conclusion that this need would not be met when someone has become homeless, has been exiled from their home. Many of us have this need met, with a warm comfortable bed and a fridge full of food so it may be difficult to understand the hardship of not having this basic need fulfilled.

When our basic need is met, we move up to our safety need. For many of us, we feel safe in our homes. We can lock our doors and there is no impending danger while we reside at home within a safe community. For others, homelife is uncertain or even abusive, therefore producing a feeling of lack of safety and discomfortable, creating great stress in a person's life.

Only after these two needs are met, can we move up to one of the most powerful needs, the need to be loved and to love. What many do not understand is that love requires self-love, in order for love to be fully expressed. Self-love serves as a form of protection as it leads us to making decisions that are in our best interest. When we love ourselves unconditionally, despite our imperfections, we are less likely to put ourselves in situations where people criticize us or mistreat us. Sometimes students who feel unloved will seek to fulfill this need by acting out in the classroom. If you're bereft of love, any attention is nourishing, even if it's negative attention.

The next need, self-esteem, can only be considered once we have fulfilled our need for love. This is an extremely important point as we too often try to teach individuals self-esteem before they have love of self. This particular level can cause a lot of trauma for the student as they seek to fulfill this emptiness in unhealthy ways, like through substances, food, oppositional behavior, sex, gaming etc.

It is imperative to teach students how to love and approve of themselves so that they may rise toward esteem. The exercises throughout this cognitive therapy section are designed to give students a better understanding of self and to show them that their greatest fan has to be themselves.

We want to be recognized by others and feel a sense of importance. This is why students will affiliate with different clubs and teams striving for social recognition. If there are none that suit their interests, they may turn to negative groups or gangs to fulfill this longing to belong.

The last need is self-actualization, the need to pursue one's highest potential. For many students, this will be difficult to conceive as they have yet to discover their passion or core interests. Self-actualization can be achieved in many ways, by reaching a life goal such as certain grade GPA, or becoming proficient at an instrument, or an art form, or attaining high levels of career success. For many, this could also be realized by becoming a parent later in life. Many who fail to meet the love need or the self-esteem need, might never recognize that self-actualization has actually occurred. For example, a driven stock broker who becomes a workaholic as a way to fill a love void, may achieve great prosperity, but lacking self-love, he is unable to truly feel the glory of his achievement.

According to Maslow, people who have achieved self-actualization possess the following qualities:

- They communicate truthfully and honestly
- They strive for goodness
- They feel a sense of interconnectedness with others and with life
- They demonstrate aliveness and spontaneity
- They trust ever-changing nature of life
- They seek justice, equality and inclusivity
- They don't stress, they live with ease
- They are independent and self-sufficient
- They are playful and full of joy and awe

Does this list look similar to that of a mindfulness practitioner?

We begin with this lesson so that students can gain a better understanding of what is motivating their behavior. Students are less likely to have outbursts in the classroom once they realize their behaviour reflects an unfulfilled need and others are there to witness it. They are instead, more inclined to seek appropriate help to fulfill the unmet need in a healthier manner.

What a person can be, s/he must be. This need we call self-actualization.

Abraham Maslow

EXERCISE HAND-OUT: THE NEEDS CHART - WHERE DO YOU FIT?

In order to be fulfilled, it is important to understand how much of each need we require in our lives. If you understand these needs and how important they are in your life, you can find fulfilling ways to satisfy them.

The following chart outlines the schematic of needs.

Survival	Safety	Love & belonging	Self-esteem	Self-actualization
Physiological needs of food, clothing, shelter	Refuge from harm, freedom from danger	Relational connection with self and others	Regard for self and social recognition	Fulfillment of one's life goals

EXERCISE: FULFILMENT OF NEEDS

Objective

To identify who and what is meeting your needs and to what extent.

Instructions

Within each circle, write down the name of each need inside the circle and then write around it, the names of family members, friends, teammates and things that help you to meet each individual need.

On a scale of one to five (1-5), five being the highest, rate how much each need is being satisfied in your life

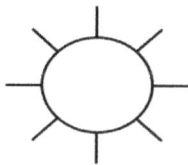

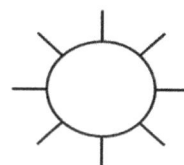

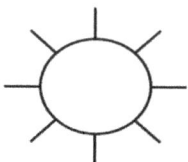

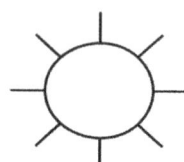

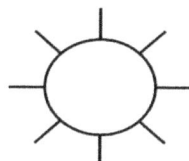

For example, my needs are as follows:

Survival	Safety	Love & belonging	Self-esteem	Self-actualization
5	5	3	2	2

Place your score in the boxes below

Survival	Safety	Love & belonging	Self-esteem	Self-actualization

After reflecting on your results, choose one need to focus on right now:

What steps can you take to boost the fulfillment of this need?

Record your actions and the results or improvements that followed and note any changes in other needs as well.

EXERCISE: ROOM OF YOUR INNER-SELF VISUALIZATION

The following will describe a process called "room of your inner-self visualization." This can be beneficial for those who come from extremely dysfunctional/co-dependent backgrounds Although our needs are present (survival, safety, love/belonging, esteem and actualization), we can lose the ability to hear the voice of each need This technique will help us to clarify our needs.

Introduction

For many of us, due to the dysfunction in our lives, it is difficult to remain quiet and hear our inner voices Whenever we face a decision, we hear a number of voices—our parents, friends, children, partners, bosses, etc. All of these voices are coming at us, repeating their messages in our mind Some messages are self-serving, wanting us to do what is best for them, not us. Some are coming from the pain of dysfunction, such as alcoholism.

We must stay in tune with our own inner voice. The voice that tells us when there is danger, when something is just not right, and when something is good for us.

Although it can be difficult to hear this inner voice, there is an exercise designed to get you in touch with this beacon on the winding road; the voice that has been suppressed over the years; the one that you have disassociated with as you react to people telling you to do things their way.

Children, as well as those in dysfunctional families, suppress their ability to hear their inner voice This is because the negative family structure teaches them not to feel, think, or react.

An example of this would be a home that has a mother who experiences challenges with alcoholism The child knows that there is a problem with the mother as she passes out all the time, but the father, in denial, declares there is no problem He exclaims to everyone that his wife does not have a drinking problem; that she is just under a lot of pressure The child learns not to trust what he sees, thinks, or feels He denies his own voice over that of his father.

This can also happen with teenagers as their peers struggle for control over them They do not feel right about doing something, but their own inner voice is drowned out by the insistence of friends. We drown out our own inner voice, saying that it is not okay to smoke because we hear our peers' voices saying, "Do this and we will accept you."

Objective

The following exercise will help you to get in touch with this inner voice. You can use this exercise whenever you are having difficulty making a decision or want to get in touch with your needs.

Instructions and Script

The following relaxation exercise is one of the most effective I have ever experienced Using soft music can enhance this process, but it is not necessary.

Find a comfortable space, and if possible, lie flat on your back If not possible, sit in a comfortable position with legs uncrossed.

With eyes closed, breathe gently into your belly Focus your energy on the breath as it slowly lifts the belly out as you breathe in and down as you breathe out Continue to do this for a few moments.

Now, focus your energy on your feet As you breathe in, tighten your toes as tight as it feels comfortable, and as you breathe out, let go Breathe in again and tighten your calf muscles Let go as you breathe out. Continue this process with the thighs, buttocks, stomach, chest, hands, neck, face and scalp Pause for a few seconds in between one group of muscles and the next.

Now, tighten every muscle in your body as tight as you can—breathe in as you tighten the muscles—breathe out as you let go.

In order to go deeper into relaxation, visualize an escalator in front of you, and on the count of 10 step onto the escalator.

10. on the count of 10, step on the escalator, and go deeper and deeper in to relaxation
9. feel your body going down as the escalator goes down
8. you are becoming more and more relaxed
7. your body is one with the escalator; the further it goes down, the deeper you become relaxed
6. you are going further and further down the escalator
5. there is nothing to do nothing to become, just go further into relaxation
4. deeper and deeper
3. you see the bottom of the escalator ahead
2. you feel completely relaxed
1. step off the escalator

Now your body is totally relaxed You can remain in this position for as long as you feel comfortable There is nothing to do, nothing to become.

With your mind's eye, picture a hallway leading to a magnificent door This doorway leads to the room of your inner self A place for you to be with you No one else can come into this room, for this room is just a place for you.

Notice the detail of the door, the type of wood and handle Are there any designs in the wood? Remember that this door leads to your inner room—a place for you to be with you Open the door and walk into the room.

This is the room of your inner self—a place for you to go when the world is just becoming too hectic Notice that this room has all your favourite belongings - all your books, pictures, music, trophies - but at the same time, no living entity This room is just for you No one can come into this room, for this space is for you to be with you.

Look around the room and notice that in this room is a beautiful chair This chair was made for you and no one else Notice the detail of the chair—the intricate detail of the work that went into making this chair Sit in this chair and allow the chair to encase your body This chair is so comfortable, it allows you to become even more relaxed.

In front of this chair is a huge picture window Look out of this window and see your most favourite scene It could be the ocean It could be a field of flowers It could be a mountain area –whatever you find the most relaxing Hold that vision now and allow it to help you in relaxing further Sit here and take in his magnificent scene Take in the comfort of this room, the security of being in this room with just you This is your place. It is a space to be with just you, free from all the other voices that try to influence your decisions.

This is a time for you to hear your own voice To hear what you need to hear Ask yourself, "What is it that I need now, at this point in my life?" Listen for the answer If the answer does not come, ask again Tell yourself you will meet that need and will try to listen to your inner voice on a daily basis.

If you have a decision to make, you can also ask your inner voice for guidance Listen to your voice and hear what you need to do in order to make that decision Remember that any time you need to be alone or hear your inner voice, you can come here to be with you.

Get up out of the chair and look around the room See all of your favourite objects in this room Remember this space, for this is your place to be with you Walk toward the door Open the door and leave the room feeling peaceful and secure in the knowledge that you have this hidden sanctuary Close the door as you leave Remember that you can come back here any time.

Coming back to the awareness of being in the present moment, open your eyes, feeling refreshed and relaxed.

After reflecting on your "Inner Room" experience:

1. Write about the experience. It could be in written paragraphs, words, poems, sketching- whatever suits your style of expression.

_____

_____

_____

_____

2. Include what it was you said you needed.

_____

_____

_____

3. After completing the writing exercise about your experience, re-read what you wrote and ask yourself: "What do I need in order to satisfy my need?" Write your answers below.

_____

_____

_____

_____

EXERCISE: CLEARING

What happens when we constantly try to achieve a goal that seems to be elusive?

There are times when our deep negative beliefs about ourselves are so ingrained they deter our achievements These doubts sit in our subconscious, sending subliminal messages that we are just not good enough.

To help get in touch with self-destructive, negative voices, many therapists use a process called *clearing* By getting in touch and letting go of the negative voices, we are free to accept what has been out of reach because of thoughts such as, "I will never..."

Objective

To get in touch with self-destructive, negative voices that prevent us from reaching goals.

Instructions

Use one blank page of paper.

Follow the process outlined below.

Step 1: Write a Goal

At the top of the page, write a goal that you have struggled to obtain; one that you have made numerous attempts to achieve and yet you seem to always fall short Your mind says, "I will never get there, maybe it's not for me."

Step 2: Free-write

This is a constant stream of thoughts that you write down without lifting the pen from the paper. You will continue for an extended period of time You will put down every reason you feel this goal is not attainable No matter how stupid it seems, include it on the paper Do not think about what you are writing, just let it flow The length of time can be anywhere between 5 minutes and a half an hour.

Step 3: Read and Tate

After you have stopped writing, read everything you have written As you are reading, realize that this is a story and there are elements of this story that have more power over you than others When something speaks to you such as a statement "I am too stupid," put a star next to it, the more it speaks to you, the more stars you write You are rating the story and the negative beliefs that force you from going forward When you finish rating them, choose one. Write it on a separate piece of paper.

Step 4: Positive Statement

Transform this one belief into a positive statement. For example, if you want to be a public speaker and your strongest core negative belief is that you are "too stupid", re-write this statement as "I am an intelligent person with something to say that people want to hear". Your initial reaction to this exercise might be to think this is a lie, however *the lie is that you cannot achieve this goal.*

Everyone is intelligent; everyone has gifts as a child. Somehow you picked up that your speaking ability was not at an appropriate level That is the lie Let go of the lie.

EMPOWERED ACTION

However dysfunctional my family was, both my mother and father taught me one thing: no matter how bad life gets (in most cases) you still have choice as to how to live your life My mother lived with lupus for 18 years, despite her doctors giving her four years to live She had a strong will to live and the year she died, only weighing 78 pounds, she attended the New Year's Ball She chose to not allow the disease to control her life and exercised that way of living as much as her body would allow. Regardless of how we feel physically or mentally, we always have some degree of power over what we do and how we live.

FOUR COMPONENTS OF BEHAVIOR

Cognitive therapy, as defined in this manual, is comprised of four components of behaviour.

The first one is DOING, which would be any physical task that we are engaged in at a given time, be it playing tennis or resting in a chair.

The next one is THINKING, which includes focused thoughts that occur when we're concentrating on a task as well as random thoughts that occur when the mind is idle or dreaming.

The next one is FELLINGS, which are emotional states or reactions, such as anger or joy. Some feelings are readily apparent to those around us and other times, we conceal them to hide pain or sadness.

Finally we have BODY TALK: our bodies expressions reflect our thoughts and feelings, for example, if I have a thought that I am unprepared for an exam or interview, I may feel an ache in my stomach.

From the information provided above, we can see how all four components work in the above situation Although she was physically ill, she chose to take positive action She couldn't change the fact that her body was dying but she could choose her thoughts and her actions She recounted many times that she was "not going to sit around being depressed, waiting to die".

If we mindfully choose our thoughts and actions, in many cases, feelings and body talk will change. For example, countless studies indicate that people who exercise have less severe periods of depression than people who don't exercise While participating in an activity, such as playing tennis, we are less likely to think negative thoughts. Therefore, we create more positive feelings and diminish the negative effects of stress on the body.

When students fail tests, they may start to think they are failures and do nothing but sit around and mope, which manifests into feelings of depression which physically may develop into sluggishness.

That being said, we cannot avoid pain and control every facet of life As a wise teacher once asked, "If we were always happy, how would we ever recognize it when we were?" We must experience the lows of life in order to appreciate the highs.

With the high rates of depression and suicide, it is evident that students understand what it means to be low Understanding how to work with our thoughts and actions provide students with a strategy for creating wellbeing, without using non-prescribed substances that simply numb our feelings.

A brief note on drugs: In some cases, the best course of treatment for a mental illness or chemical imbalance is prescription drugs, however, studies have shown that cognitive therapy with prescription drugs is more effective than the use drugs alone.

EXERCISE: PUTTING THE FOUR COMPONENTS OF BEHAVIOR INTO ACTION

This exercise is designed to help you look at a current situation and analyze it from the perspective of the four components of behavior.

How do you get what you want? All anyone can do is use their behaviours. *The four components of behaviour* (feelings, thinking, doing and body talk or physical symptoms) can be exercised when wanting to achieve a certain outcome.

Consider a recent situation in your life in which you were attempting to get a need met (like trying out for a team). Describe it briefly here:

_____

_____

_____

_____

_____

_____

_____

_____

_____

Now, list some behaviors you used during the situation.

FEELINGS Example: excitement.	THINKING Example: Worry.

ACTING OR DOING Example: best effort	BODY TALK (physical symptoms) examples: sweating, knees shaking

After doing this exercise, you begin to realize a very important aspect of life We have no control over our feelings and body talk but we do have power over what we <u>think</u> and <u>do</u> Feelings and body talk occur in direct relation to what we are thinking and doing.

For example, if I was anxious about an exam, worrying causes me to feel fear and I have pains in my gut If I can learn to turn my thinking away from a negative perspective about the exam, the feelings of fear will be replaced with confidence and the stomach ache will be replaced with energy. I direct my thoughts by thinking in terms of solutions, and I seek the appropriate help to pass the exam.

EXERCISE: MATCHING REAL WORLD WITH IDEAL WORLD

Objective

To identify the difference between your real world and your ideal world and learn ways to manage your feelings as you move toward your ideal world.

There is a real world and there is an ideal world picture of what you want for your life When these pictures do not match, we can be flooded with frustration or even hopelessness and run the risk of abandoning our dreams. But with discipline and hard work, we can fuse these two realities into one.

Describe a real-world situation in your life that does not match the picture of what you want in your ideal world.

_____

_____

_____

_____

_____

1. What are your feelings when the scenarios don't match?

_____

_____

_____

_____

2. Do you have any physical symptoms? What is your body talk (how does your body feel)?

_____

_____

_____

_____

3. What are you thinking about when your pictures don't match?

_____

_____

_____

_____

4. What are your actions? What are you doing?

_____

_____

_____

_____

5. Now decide, are your actions helping you? Write about it in the space provided below.

_____

_____

_____

_____

EXERCISE: IS THE VISION FOR YOUR IDEAL WORLD REALISTIC?

How do you know if your vision for your ideal world is reasonable? Has this picture been in your mind for a long time? Does it seem that no matter what you do, you cannot achieve it? If you answered yes, this could be a clue that your goal might be unattainable or impossible given the fixed (unchangeable) details of your life. For example, there are only a certain few who meet the stringent physical requirements to be a jockey, or a model. Many teens today strive for celebrity status because that is what our culture presents as successful, which is unrealistic for most people. The reality of being a celebrity involves more than just the glamour and ease that's presented to the world. The lives of celebrities are wrought with pressure, paparazzi and expectations.

Success is an interesting word that means different things to different people. Before jumping into crystalizing your vision of success, you might want to consider how you've been conditioned to define success in our culture. Today's version of success is largely oriented around money, climbing the corporate ladder and winning. You can question this view by asking yourself:

- What truly makes me happy?
- When do I feel most fulfilled?
- What do I long to leave behind when my time is up?
- What skills do I need to develop in order to fulfill this dream?

Your answers to these questions will help to clarify what success means to you, which can guide your next steps.

It may be helpful to consider how long you want to keep striving for a dream (and perhaps living in frustration about a dream that is impossible, or seemingly impossible). Remember, at any time you can redefine your vision to make your dream more attainable. This more reasonable ideal world might lead to more contentment, but it may also lead you in the direction of your ultimate goal. With any dream, it's helpful to break it down into incremental steps and work to achieve one thing at a time. As life unfolds, you may realize as you grow older and wiser, that your initial dream wasn't truly aligned with your life goals anyway. As Garth Brooks once sang "Sometimes God's greatest gifts are unanswered prayers."

Write about a desire you have for your ideal world that you believe might be an unrealistic dream. Then, think of ways you can revise the goal to get what you want Write about the revised vision in the space below.

My unrealistic vision is:

_____

_____

_____

_____

_____

The revised vision is:

_____

_____

_____

_____

_____

_____

Once you have finished your revised picture, go to the next exercise on "EAST" Goals and apply your revised picture.

EXERCISE: A ROAD MAP FOR REACHING A GOAL

The E.A.S.T process helps us to mindfully set a goal and then, just as the sun rises from the east, encourages us to view each day as a new beginning. The following exercise is a step by step process that helps you create the life of your dreams, aligned with your passion.

Having a plan of action that has a high likelihood of success is the same as having a good road map for moving from one place to another. In this case, we are moving from our current state (real world) to a new desired state (ideal world). A good plan of action, like a good road map, will help you take the most direct route to get you what you want.

1st-Think of something you want but so far have not been able to achieve it

2nd-Use the following formula to write a plan of action. Try a route on your road map that you have never tried before.

_____

_____

Use the following formula to write a plan of action. Try a route on your road map that you have never tried before.

EAST Goal Formula

E - Be Exact	Indicate what the goal is, who will help, where it will happen, and how you plan to accomplish it.
A - Make it Authentic	Be true to yourself and create goals that reflect your deepest desires, which will inspire you to follow through.
S - Be Straightforward and Simple	Create a goal that you can do independently. Make it "something to do, not something to stop doing."
T – Make it Timely	Plan something you can start right away and work on it often.

	My plan
E - Be Exact	
A – Authentic	
S - Straightforward and Simple	
T - Timely	

EXERCISE: ALIGNING DESIRES AND ACTIONS WITH THE OUTCOME USING CT PRINCIPLES

Once you clarify your desire, what it is you want to attain, it's essential that you chart a course of action that will support your success. In other words, in order to achieve a desired outcome, you need to align your actions with your thoughts and feelings.

Student reflections:

What do I desire? Is what I want reasonable and possible?

_____

_____

_____

_____

_____

What is my roadmap or action plan for attaining what I want?

_____

_____

_____

_____

_____

What actions am I taking?

_____

_____

_____

_____

_____

Is what I am doing moving me toward or away from my goal?

_____

_____

_____

_____

_____

I tried my plan How did it work?

_____

_____

_____

_____

_____

EXERCISE: THE BLAME GAME

Whenever things don't go our way, or when we make a mistake, our first instinct is to blame someone else. Statements such as these are familiar to most, "He made me do it!" or "She started it by calling me a name". The Blame Game may seem like the easiest option in the moment because it's the fastest route out of a potentially shameful situation. But shirking responsibility puts us in a victim stance where life is happening to us and stealing our power to grow.

The truth is that other people's behaviour does not control our lives, our behavior does. We are fully responsible for what we choose to do and don't do. Initially this can be a difficult truth to accept because it puts us in the driver seat, but it's the only way to fully claim our power to live our own lives. By taking responsibility for our behavior, we are given the opportunity to move beyond old limiting scripts, to work hard for what we want and to move forward in a chosen direction.

Once we gain the awareness that we are ultimately responsible for everything we do and that we have the power to choose our own behaviours, we can then act consciously and more thoughtfully, instead of unconsciously and carelessly.

In this space, describe something that happened in your life, that you believe was someone else's fault.

_____

_____

_____

_____

_____

Now reflect on your description and see if you can identify in the space below where you were at least partially responsible.

_____

_____

_____

_____

_____

EXERCISE: LIFE, DEATH, LIFE

All relationships follow a cyclical pattern of life, death, life. We meet someone that we feel emotionally connected to and we enter into relationship, be it friendship or otherwise. This is a life phase. Then, as some time passes, conflicts arise and we question the relationship. We react out of hurt or anger, mistakenly assuming that it's not working out and choose to end things.

It is during this death phase, that we can use a few cognitive therapy practices to help move into a life phase again. Having a courageous conversation about each other's needs, or non-negotiables, can help both parties feel safe again within the container of the relationship. Some examples of needs might be: confidentiality, respect for boundaries and honest communication.

Personal Responsibility

The situation can be unpacked by both people taking turns to bravely identify who owns what part of the interaction. Simply stating our needs and claiming personal responsibility for our part of the death phase may, in many cases, resolve the issues and re-ignite the connection (the Blame Game exercise can also help here). We can then move into another life phase.

If further work is required, move onto the following exercise:

Needs and Non-negotiables

The strategy for identifying each other's needs can go as follows: each individual can write down what they need in a relationship. Below that they write what is non-negotiable (what they cannot compromise on, such as trust). Each person then explains how to ideally meet these needs. For example, I may need positive energy first thing in the morning, and so I can request that conversations be uplifting at breakfast.

Sharing of Needs

Then both parties can come together and invite each person to read off their needs, highlighting their non-negotiables. If the other person is amenable to the requests and can agree to meeting these needs, then the relationship may have a new foundation with which to begin again.

Action Steps

The true test is for each person to put their commitments into action, by actually doing what was discussed and agreed upon. If each person's needs are consistently honored, the relationship has a good likelihood of continuing with an ever-stronger connection.

*It's important to be aware that some of us, hold onto relationships when they should actually die because they are not healthy for us and they don't help us to thrive in life. If the health of the relationship is in question, one can do further research on co-dependency to help sift through the issues and clarify what's really going on.

1. My needs in a relationship are:

_____

_____

_____

_____

_____

2. What is non-negotiable?

_____

_____

_____

_____

_____

3. The best way to meet these needs are:

_____

_____

_____

_____

_____

4. Action plan:

_____

_____

_____

_____

_____

Student Reflections

- Think of a relationship in your past where you experienced the beginning life phase, followed by a death phase and you ended the relationship, perhaps prematurely.
- On the contrary, reflect on a relationship that was unhealthy and needed to die but you kept it alive anyway?

WHY DO WE CHOOSE MISERY?

It can be very difficult for us to face the fact that we choose most of the misery we experience. Let's consider a student who has failed to pass a test. Most student have options available to them, such as getting extra help (doing) and working hard to study the material. Instead, he may choose to be depressed and tell himself that he will never pass the course. The choice to "do nothing" may be a way of avoiding feelings of sadness, insecurity, or anxiety. But this approach does not line up with his vision for graduating, it only causes more misery and affirms his lack of belief in himself.

Students may also choose misery in relationships. Grief is an essential and healthy process to go through when we've experienced a loss of any kind, including the loss of a relationship. But if we linger too long in a grief pattern, it can mature into a chronic state of depression. At this point we can choose to stay low or choose to mobilize our energy with uplifting thoughts, influences, activities and conversations, which will help to turn the tide on depression.

To heal from a loss, a student can participate in positive activities, such as spending time with friends, trying something new, or volunteering This is doing. Instead of doing something positive, however, many people dwell in their feelings of sadness, which is destructive long term.

- What are some reasons why people might choose misery?
- The following are a few suggestions
- as a way of getting love and attention
- to avoid examining deeper feelings, like rejection
- to control others and maintain their affection
- to avoid failure
- What other reasons do you think people choose misery, whether consciously or unconsciously?

EXERCISE: EXPLORING YOUR REASONS FOR CHOOSING MISERY

In the space provided, free write (without judgment) about a time in your life when you chose misery, (sorrow that exceeded the natural grieving or sadness period).

_____

_____

_____

_____

_____

With your new understanding of misery, what other behaviours could you employ in the future when faced with a similar situation?

_____

_____

_____

_____

_____

CHOOSING TO THINK POSITIVELY ABOUT OURSELVES

Sometimes we may choose misery because we have developed a habit of negative self-talk Negative self-talk refers to the (often recurring) negative thoughts that flow through our minds about ourselves Some examples of negative self-talk are

1. I am so boring, no wonder no one is sitting with me.
2. I'm destined for poor grades because I never get my work done on time.
3. Who could ever love someone who looks like me?

As we grow in awareness of how to live more mindfully, we realize that our thoughts are not always truthful or accurate and therefore, can't always be trusted When we worry or ruminate about something, we have the choice to turn our minds from these negative thoughts toward more helpful thought patterns. The following exercises are designed to empower us to let go of self-defeating thoughts and cultivate more positive mind states.

EXERCISE: SELF-ESTEEM LIST

It is very easy to recognize the positive qualities of others, but sometimes it is hard to see them in ourselves We all have positive attributes and yet we fail to acknowledge them We constantly reminded our students to offer themselves loving thoughts whenever they walked by a mirror, by saying something kind about themselves. It could be as simple as repeating the statement, "I love you just the way you are."

With the unrealistic beauty standards that we are all affected by today, it is all too easy to tear ourselves apart with criticism one body part at a time. The effects of self-criticism can run deep and last a lifetime, destroying our confidence and our self-esteem. Starting today, you are invited to take a stand against such self-destruction and commit to changing your perspective by noticing aspects of yourself that you can appreciate.

Let's get more detailed by exploring the various aspects of yourself that are nothing short of amazing Note that if you get stumped (a reflection that you're being stingy with yourself), try imagining what your parents, or other loved one's might say about you.

We'll start with your body by asking yourself what parts of your body you can appreciate. What do these body parts enable you to do and experience?

_____

_____

_____

What aspects of your personality do you appreciate? (non-value based qualities as taught in the art therapy classes in this manual, such as kindness, hard-working, trustworthy etc).

_____

_____

_____

What do you appreciate about your talents, your interests?

_____

_____

_____

To summarize this important exercise, it's helpful to create positive statements that reflect the things you appreciate about yourself, for example:

1. I acknowledge that I am very generous.
2. I love my healthy hair.
3. I love how I make people laugh.
4. I appreciate that I am a great problem solver.
5. I enjoy being a powerful activist for change.

Can you create a list of ten things from the reflections above?

1.

2.

3.

4.

5.

6.

7.

8.

9.

10.

What distinguishes faith in ourselves from conceit is the fact that conceit lays claim
to specialness, but our fundamental nature is not personal, it's universal, it's shared

Sharon Salzberg

EXERCISE: CELEBRATING SUCCESS

Objective

Celebrate successes and recognize accomplishments.

Our fast-paced, productivity-obsessed society teaches us to work hard and strive to accomplish - but it skips a very important part of the whole process, which is to take time at the end of a project (and before you start another) to celebrate our achievements. Whenever we push our growing edge or try something new or bring an idea to fruition, or succeed at a challenge, it is cause for celebration!

This exercise is designed to teach us how to celebrate our successes, without judging their worthiness based on their scale, or importance in the world. Sometimes we have to walk before we can run, so give yourself the freedom to start small to familiarize your mind with this frame of thinking and then build on your successes from there. Soon you'll be noticing achievements that you make each and every day!

For example:

1. I received my driver's licence last week.
2. I speak fluent French and English.
3. I prepared a nutritious meal for the family yesterday.
4. am a reliable babysitter and earn my own money.
5. I am a skilled graphic artist.

My successes in the last month are:

_____

_____

_____

_____

_____

EXERCISE: SELF-APPRECIATION LIST

It is so easy to do for others and, at times, so hard to do for ourselves We are conditioned as young children that doing too much for oneself is selfish Although this can be true, we are largely a culture who has difficulty with self-care and appreciation.

Caring for yourself is one of the first steps to healing the body and mind disconnect by fostering inner peace and harmony.

Instructions

Create a list of the different ways you can appreciate yourself and then make a simple plan to carry out each action.

For example:

Things I can do to show appreciation for myself:	My plan for following through:
Visit friends who appreciate me	Call Olivia and invite her out for a walk
Eat something healthy	Use up the apples, kale, raisins, and spinach to make a salad for my snack instead of chips.
Buy myself my favorite flowers	Next time I'm at the store I'll pick up a bundle.

Your appreciation list and action plan:

Things I can do to show appreciation for myself:	My plan for following through:

CELEBRATION OF SELF—21 DAY CHALLENGE

This exercise, called Celebration of Self, is a valuable practice to introduce near the beginning of a mindfulness program. By spending time each day appreciating themselves, this exercise encourages students to begin relating to themselves with kindness and respect. The hope is that this practice will help to ease our children's obsession with celebrity idolization, by turning at least some of that affection onto themselves. Imagine if they spent the same amount of time on self-love as they do on social media, enviously following the lives of celebrities?

For some, it's easier to accept love from others than it is to accept love from themselves. But it's possible to change that, and it's well worth the effort since life with self-love is life lived in full color.

Here's the invitation; since it takes about 21 days to introduce a new habit, the class can commit to practicing Celebration of Self each day. According to the European Journal of Social Psychology, it takes on average 66 days to solidify a new habit, so as students successfully complete the 21-day challenge, they may feel inspired to keep going until this practice becomes a part of their daily routine.

The following are steps for the Celebration of Self practice:

- Create time in your schedule to start your day with several minutes of this practice.
- Find a designated quiet corner of your living space and fill a shelf or side table with the following items: a non-scented candle, flowers or a plant, a photo of yourself, a journal and any other items that are special to you.
- Choose one or two positive affirmation statements that inspire and reassure you. A few examples are:
  - I love and accept myself just the way I am
  - Without having to change anything, I am lovable right now
  - Today, I choose to appreciate my natural beauty
  - I give thanks for my innate gifts and talents that I've been given
  - Thank you for my life—I am blessed
- Each morning upon waking, light your candle and take a few calming breaths to arrive in your body and in the moment.
- Look at your photo and recite your affirmations slowly, feeling the words land in the deepest part of your being.
- Water your plant or flower and absorb its beauty, fragrance and life force.
- If time allows, write your reflections in a journal each day, recording how you feel about yourself and any changes or improvements that occur.

You might be wondering if this practice will foster conceit but rest assured that you are not placing yourself at a greater importance than anyone else, but simply realizing that you are a unique individual, equally worthy of love and respect. After all, the most important person who needs to believe in you, is you! Over time, if done consistently, this practice will give you an enhanced sense of self, and when that happens, your life will change.

MINDFULNESS IN SCHOOLS MANUAL

Your life is made up of the little things you do and think each day. As Mahatma Gandhi once said:

Your beliefs become your thoughts,
Your thoughts become your words,
Your words become your actions,
Your actions become your habits,
Your habits become your values,
Your values become your destiny.

CAPTURING THE MOMENT

For so many of us raised this culture, expressing our true feelings and affection to people we care about is a very scary thing. But life is uncertain, and death is a guarantee. The following is an exercise that encourages us to share our love with those we care most about.

For a former student Joseph, this exercise couldn't have come at a better time. When he was in his final year of high school, one of our students, named Joseph was given the assignment of making a list of three people whom they love. They were then encouraged to reach out to the people on their list and tell each one that they loved them. A simple act, but a really big deal, especially for this Italian boy who had never exchanged such words with his dad.

On the day the assignment was due, Joseph's dad drove him to school. As he stepped out of the car, Joseph leaned back in and said nervously "Dad, I just want you to know that I love you." To his surprise, his dad replied sheepishly, "Uh...wow...you know son, I love you too." Joseph walked into the school with tears in his eyes, never believing he'd ever have such a tender exchange with his very reserved father. He was even more grateful that he'd risked everything and said what he said because shortly thereafter, his father died suddenly of a severe heart attack.

What three people in your life would you choose to express love to?

Here's the process:

- Make a list of three people you feel incomplete with, people in your life currently or from your past whom you believe to have things left unsaid between you. Let's be clear, the intent of this assignment is to express love, not grievances, that's another assignment☺.

- Devise a plan to contact each person, be it by phone, email or in person and set a contact date to ensure you take action.

- Rehearse what you intend to say, for example "Hi Mary, I'm calling because I have been thinking about you lately. I want you to know how important you are to me and how much I appreciate your support and friendship." Simple, short and potentially transformative for your relationship.

- Remember that this is NOT an opportunity to vent your disappointments, nor is it a chance to rekindle an old flame or strive for a family inheritance. You are to approach this without expectations, detached from receiving anything in return. Just stay present to your intent and know that you're contributing to the good of the world and likely leaving a huge impact on your people's lives for being brave enough to express your love and affection.

- This may feel so rewarding and liberating that you continue to do this exercise with all of your love relationships!

POSITIVE BELIEFS

Just before you fall asleep and as soon as you wake up, your subconscious mind (theta brain wave state) is most available Have you ever noticed that as you drift off you seem to be in two different states? You can hear what is going on around you and, at the same time, you are starting to dream Have you also noticed that upon waking you initially remember your dream, and then a short time later the dream has all but disappeared? That's because the subconscious mind is most accessible in the state between sleep and wakefulness.

The subconscious mind, where our core negative beliefs reside, speaks to us all day, reciting past failures and reminding us of our limitations Therefore, in order to grow and evolve into our highest potential (see Maslow's lesson), we must learn to replace them with more supportive, positive beliefs.

We can never erase a traumatic, shameful or embarrassing experience from our past but we can over-lap the negative event with positive truths about ourselves.

One way to do this is to take your positive statement from the previous self-esteem list, write it on pieces of paper (or on your screen saver) and place it throughout the house where you will see it on a continuous basis. Every time you see it, recite it, take a breath in and let yourself absorb it.

If a negative statement arises, firmly recite to yourself, "That does not belong here" and repeat your positive statement. Additionally, as a way of feeding the sub-conscious mind, keep your positive statement by your bedside and recite it ten times or more just before you go to sleep at night and again as soon as you wake up in the morning.

SUBCONSCIOUS RE-PROGRAMMING

From the time we were born, every event, whether it has been a success or a failure, has been recorded in the subconscious mind. Our mind stores movie reels that are being played back constantly.

Some believe that the subconscious makes up 85% of the mind It is that part of the mind that speaks to us on a continuous basis. It subliminally calls upon the movies of the past that re-enforce beliefs in present time. There is a way to access this part of our brain and insert new reels that over-lap the old ones. It is referred to as *subconscious re-programming*.

Writing exams is a common fear shared among many students. No matter how prepared they are, some students freeze when the exam is put in front of them. The subconscious speaks to them and blocks information by sending them into a fight or flight reaction which makes our thinking mind inaccessible.

Even the memory of the event can cause the same physical symptoms. This is one feature of Post-Traumatic Stress Disorder. What we want to do is insert positive memories that will have a stronger influence than the negative ones. To be successful, we must replace the negative or stressful memories of writing the exam with images and thoughts of successfully completing the exam into the subconscious mind. The student must visualize themselves writing easefully with ideas and answers flowing freely.

EXERCISE DEALING WITH FEAR IN THE SUBCONSCIOUS

Objective

The following exercise will help anyone deal with a specific fear.

Part 1

Write a script about overcoming a fear such as an exam. The script should be in the present tense and express the good feelings you feel as you write free of fear.

Bring all of your senses in to the writing of the script, sight, taste, smell, touch and hearing.

Visualize yourself writing the exam in a calm and confident manner and then walking out of the room feeling proud, self-assured and excited about successfully completing this endeavour.

This should be read at least twice a day.

Part 2

Accessing the subconscious

In order to access the subconscious mind, we have to drop into a relaxed state. The following exercise is an effective teaching script for leading someone into a state of relaxation, which can be done with soft instrumental music.

Settle into the moment, resting here in a comfortable position. Invite your breath to slow down and deepen. Soft, smooth deep breaths.

In order to go deeper into relaxation, visualize an escalator in front of you, and on the count of 10 step onto the escalator.

10. on the count of 10, step on the escalator, and go deeper and deeper in to relaxation
9. feel your body going down as the escalator goes down
8. you are becoming more and more relaxed
7. your body is one with the escalator; the further it goes down, the deeper you become relaxed
6. you are going further and further down the escalator
5. there is nothing to do nothing to become, just go further into relaxation
4. deeper and deeper
3. you see the bottom of the escalator
2. you feel completely relaxed
1. step off the escalator

After completing the relaxation exercise: remember the script you wrote and visualize it as if it were the present moment. Live it Allow yourself to feel all the satisfaction of finally achieving your goal.

This is an optional closing, if leading this exercise in class

Come to sitting and find sankalpa mudra, the hand gesture of intention, whereby you rest right hand over left at heart center. Listen to these words and let them charge your dreams with hope and possibility:

Today, *be* the person of your dreams.
See life through their eyes.
Make decisions with their mind
Let every thought, word, feeling and action
come from their perspective,
as if you've already arrived.
Today, say yes to the best that is within you!

Pillar 4
Story Telling

Since the beginning of time people have used stories as a means for teaching and passing on wisdom. People have an inherent love for being read or told stories as they engender feelings of magic and wonder, awakening our imagination.

Instead of demanding the intellectual mind to memorize information, story-telling taps into the emotional aspect of the brain, leaving deep memories of the feelings experienced through the stories It improves listening and communication skills, while sharpening social and emotional intelligences.

Story telling is one of the best ways to deliver any lesson, since the concept is linked to an emotion. This enables us to relate to others through our shared emotional experience, which naturally cultivates compassion and empathy.

THE STORY OF THE FIREBIRD

by Michael Meade[5]

The Story of the Firebird is helpful for teaching the concept of living in the moment. In the story, the Horse of Power will tell the Hunter, "The trouble is not now, the trouble lies before you." He conveys the message that if we allow fear of the future to consume us, we will be unable to both manage challenges and see the benefits in the present moment.

We realize that we can only do our best in this moment. We communicate the value of allowing events to unfold, in their own time. We will not neglect consequences, rather steer ourselves towards finding solutions in the present moment. We are trying learn to do what we need to in this moment, and then let go. The worry will never change the outcome.

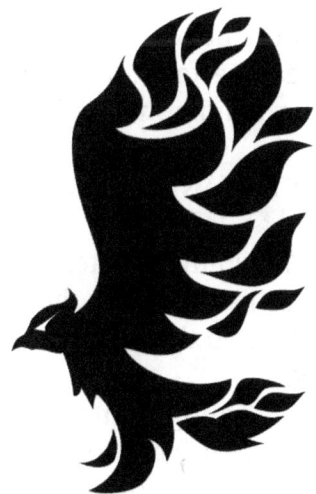

---

[5] Meade, Michael. 1994. *Men and The Water of Life: Initiation and the Tempering of Men*. San Francisco: Harper.

Once upon a time (not this time but another time), in a certain place (not this place, but another place), where broad forests stood, and many birds flew among the ancient trees, there was a realm ruled by a mighty king.

In the realm, there was a young Hunter. The Hunter had a horse that was a Horse of Power. It was such a horse as belonged to the men of long ago; a swift horse with a broad chest, eyes like fire, and hoofs of iron. There were no such horses nowadays. They sleep deeply in the earth with the men who rode them, waiting for a time when the world was in need of them again. At that time, all the great horses will thunder up from under the ground and the valiant men of old will leap from their graves.

Those men of old will ride the Horses of Power. With a swing of clubs and a thundering of hooves, they will sweep the earth clean of the enemies of God. At least, that's what my grandfather said, and his grandfather said before him, and if they don't know, who does?

One day, in springtime, a young hunter was riding through the forest on his Horse of Power. The leaves were growing green in the sun and there were little blue flowers under the trees. Squirrels ran in the branches, hares worked through the undergrowth, yet it was quiet. No birds sang. The young Hunter listened for the birds, but the forest was silent, except for the scratching of four-footed beasts, the dropping of pine cones, and the heavy stamping of the Horse of Power.

"What has happened to the birds?" the young Hunter said aloud. He had scarcely uttered the words when he noticed a big curved feather lying on the path before him. The feather was larger than that of a swan and longer than that of an eagle. It lay there glittering on the path like a flame of the sun. It was a feather of gold.

Now, the youth knew why there was no singing in the forest; the Firebird had flown that way, and the flame on the path was a feather from its burning breast.

Suddenly, the Horse of Power spoke and said, "Leave the flaming feather where it lies. If you take it you will be sorry - for you will know trouble and you will learn the meaning of fear."

The young Hunter turned the matter over in his mind. "Should I pick up the golden feather or not? I have no wish to learn fear. Who needs more trouble?" But on the other hand, if he picked the feather up and presented it to the King, the King would be pleased. He would reward and honour him, for no king had a feather from the burning breast of a firebird.

(STOP AND DISCUSS: WOULD YOU PICK UP THE FEATHER? WHY OR WHY NOT?)

The young Hunter turned the decision this way and that. The more he thought, the more he desired to carry the feather to the King. He knelt to the ground, picked up the feather, remounted the horse, and galloped back through the green forest directly to the palace of the King.

The young Hunter entered the great hall of the palace, walked its length, bowed before the King, and offered the feather as a gift. "Thank you," said the King, "a shining feather from the burning breast of the Firebird is a thing of great wonder and value. But a single feather is not a fit gift for a king. The whole bird held here before me, that would be a fitting gift! Since you have found the feather of the Firebird, you will be able to bring me the Firebird itself. Either you present the whole bird here before me, or the edge of this sword will forge a path between your chin and your shoulders."

The young Hunter bowed his head and went out weeping bitter tears, wiser now in the knowledge of what it means to be afraid. The Horse of Power was waiting and asked the youth why he was weeping. The Hunter said he was required by the King to bring him the whole firebird. Since no man could do that, he was weeping at the fate that awaited him – the certain loss of his head. The Horse didn't console him, didn't offer to flee with him, and didn't dismiss his fears.

"I told you so," said the Horse. "I said if you took the feather you would learn fear. Well, grieve no more. The trouble is not now; the trouble lies before you. Go to the King and ask that a hundred sacks of maize be emptied and scattered in the open field near the palace. Ask him for three lengths of strong rope, and to be ready by dawn.

The next day, as the red of dawn burned the darkness from the sky, the young Hunter rode out on the Horse of Power and came to the open field. He covered the ground with maize. In the centre of the field stood a great oak tree with spreading boughs. The Hunter hid himself in the branches of the tree and the Horse of Power wandered loose in the field.

The sun rose and the sky grew into gold. Suddenly, there was a noise in the forest surrounding the field. The trees shook and swayed and seemed ready to fall. A violent wind blew. In the distance, the sea piled itself into waves with crests of foam and the Firebird came flying from the other side of the world. Huge, golden and flaming in the light of the sun, it flew. Then it dropped, with open wings onto the field and began to eat the maize.

The Horse of Power wandered nearer and nearer, as the Firebird ate. Suddenly, the Horse stepped on one of its fiery wings and pressed it heavily to the ground. As the Firebird struggled, the youth tied three ropes around the bird. He hefted it over his back and mounted the Horse. In this fashion, the three rode to the King's palace.

The youth carried the great bird into the palace. The broad wings hung on either side of him, like fiery shields. As he moved through the great hall, he left a trail of flaming feathers on the floor. The King gazed on the bird with delight, thanked the youth for his services, raised him to a noble rank, and immediately charged him with another task.

"Since you have known how to bring me the Firebird, you will know how to bring me the bride I have long desired. In the Land of Never, at the very edge of the world, where the red sun rises in flame from behind the blue sea, lives the beautiful Vasilisa. It is she whom I desire. If you bring her to me, I will reward you with silver and gold. If not, my sword will pass between your head and shoulders like the wind that tears through a forest, taking off the tops of trees."

The young Hunter walked out, weeping bitter tears that fell to the floor of the great hall. He descended the steps to where the Horse of Power was waiting in the courtyard.

"Why do you weep now, master?" asked the Horse.

"Because the King has ordered me to go to the Land of Never and bring back the beautiful Vasilisa, or he'll off my head!"

"Didn't I tell you that you would know trouble?" Asked the Horse. "Well, weep no more and grieve not. The trouble is not now; the trouble lies before you. Go to the King and ask for a silver tent with a golden roof and all kinds of food and drink to take on the journey."

The youth asked, and the King gave him a silver tent with a gold embroidered roof, every kind of wine, and the tastiest of foods to take with him. The youth mounted the Horse of Power and they rode many days and many nights. They came at last to the edge of the world, where the red sun rises in flame from behind the deep sea.

The young Hunter looked out on the blue sea and there he saw the beautiful Vasilisa floating in a boat with golden oars. The youth let the Horse loose to wander and feed. As for himself, he pitched the silver tent with the golden roof at the edge of the world where the shore met the water. He set out the great variety of food and drink, dressed himself in the finest clothes, and sat down to wait for the beautiful Vasilisa.

Vasilisa spied the embroidered tent where it stood in the sand, between the green grass and the blue sea, and she admired it. She came to the shore in her silver boat. From there she could see scenes from old stories embroidered on the sides of the tent. She saw the open door of the tent and, within it, the hunter, who offered her old wine and fine foods. She accepted and they ate and talked and toasted each other.

The wine was heavy and foreign to her and her eyes closed as if the night itself had perched upon them. She fell into a deep sleep. Quickly the youth folded the tent, lifted the beautiful Vasilisa and mounted the Horse of Power. She lay as light as a feather in his arms and was not awakened by the thundering of the iron hoofs on the ground as the three of them rode back to the palace of the King.

The youth carried Vasilisa to the King and the joy of the King was great. He thanked the Hunter and rewarded him with silver and gold and, again, raised him in rank. But then Vasilisa awoke to discover that she was far from her blue sea. She began to weep and grieve. The King tried to comfort her, telling her of their upcoming marriage and that she would be queen. But his efforts were in vain for she longed to be in her boat on the blue sea.

The King insisted on the marriage and Vasilisa finally said, "In the middle of the deep sea there lies a great stone. Hidden under that stone are my wedding clothes. Unless I wear those garments, I will marry no one at all. Let him who brought me here return to that land and find my gown." The King ordered the youth to go at once, saying that if he brought the garments back, he would be rewarded; if not, his head would roll toward the sea.

The young Hunter walked out, weeping as before, and again the Horse asked for the cause of his grief. "The King has ordered me to return to the edge of the world and retrieve Vasilisa's wedding garments from beneath a great stone at the very bottom of the sea. I'll surely die attempting it and if I don't die from that, my head will roll from his sword. But there is new trouble as well. Even if I should manage to bring the wedding clothes, I'll be helping the King marry the beautiful Vasilisa and I'd rather die than see that!"

"I told you," said the Horse of Power, "if you picked up that flaming feather you would learn fear and find trouble. Well, grieve not. The trouble is not yet; the trouble lies before you. Now mount up and we'll go back."

After a short time or a long time, they arrived at the edge of the world and stopped at the shore of the sea. The Horse of Power saw a huge crab crawling on the sand at the edge of the sea. He approached the crab and suddenly stepped on it with its heavy hoof. The crab cried out, "Don't give me death! Give me life, and I will do whatever you ask."

The Horse said, "In the middle of the deep sea, under a great stone lies the wedding gown of the beautiful Vasilisa. Bring that gown to us."

The crab called in a voice heard over the wide sea. The sea became agitated and from all directions came crustaceans of all forms and sizes. The shore became covered with crabs and lobsters who gathered together. The old crab was the chief among the crustaceans. He directed them to move the stone at the bottom of the sea and bring up the wedding gown.

And so, the horde of crustaceans returned to the sea. After a time, the water was disturbed again, and out of it came thousands of crustaceans carrying the gold casket that contained the wedding gown.

The Horse of Power carried the young hunter, and the Hunter carried the casket and gown just as he had carried Vasilisa and the Firebird. Soon they arrived at the palace and the hunter once more walked the length of the great hall.

But now Vasilisa refused to marry the King unless the young Hunter was made to bathe in rapidly boiling water. The King ordered some of his servants to gather wood, make a great fire, place a large cauldron on the fire, and attend to it until the water boiled fully. Then he demanded the young hunter be thrown into the cauldron. The rest of the servants were busy preparing the palace for the royal wedding. A great feast was cooked as all of the King's people gathered.

Everything was ready at once: The water in the cauldron came to a seething boil, just as the wedding feast was finished. The hunter said to himself, "Now, this is trouble. Why did I ever pick up the flaming feather of the Firebird? Why did I not heed my horse?" Remembering the Horse of Power, he said to the King, "Presently I shall die in the heat of the fire. I only request that I may see my horse once more before my death." The King granted his last wish.

Once again the young hunter left the palace weeping tears that fell to the ground of the great hall. He descended the steps to where the Horse was waiting in the courtyard. "Why do you weep now?" asked the horse "I weep because the King has ordered that I be boiled to death in a cauldron already heated and ready. I weep because you and I will never more see the green trees pass above us and the ground disappearing beneath our feet as we race between earth and sky!"

"Fear not, weep not," said the Horse. "When they take you to the cauldron, do not hesitate; rather, run forward and leap into the water yourself!"

The hunter ascended the stairs and entered the hall. When the servants came for him, he ran forward and leapt into the seething cauldron. Twice he disappeared under the boiling waters and then he leapt out of the cauldron. The onlookers stood amazed at the sight, for not only had the youth survived but he was now more handsome than before, and he was imbued with a beautiful glow.

The King thought it a miracle and, seeing the beauty of the hunter, wanted to bathe in the boiling cauldron himself. He plunged into the seething water and was boiled to death in a moment. Afterward, he was buried.

The wedding feast was ready. The people gathered and the great hall was poised for the wedding of a King and a Queen. So, the beautiful Vasilisa celebrated the wedding feast with the Hunter. They became the rulers of the realm and lived long in love and accord.

FIREBIRD STORY: QUESTIONS AND ANSWERS

1. The shining feather represents opportunity for praise, reward, or recognition. Have you ever, like the young hunter, picked up a shining feather thinking it would bring you great rewards? Explain.
    a. What was the outcome?
2. The Horse of Power represents the Hunter's inner voice. In the beginning, the young hunter did not heed the warnings of the Horse of Power. Have you ever stopped listening to your inner voice?
    a. If so, describe when that occurred and why?
3. Reflect on a time in your life when an event caused you great pain, yet you grew and matured from the experience. Describe
4. Why is it that chasing desire is an endless cycle?

THE SWEETEST STRAWBERRY

One day a young man was walking down a path in a forest, when he noticed the bushes rustling to the left of him. He then heard something to the right of him. Within moments, a pack of wolves emerged from either side.

He started running away from the wolves, sprinting for his life, when he soon came to the edge of a cliff. Looking over his shoulder at the wolves gaining on him and then at the cliff in front of him, he thought with certainty that his life was over. Looking down over the cliff in despair, he noticed a vine stretching down to the ground below. With nothing to lose, he lowered himself to the edge and began to shimmy down the vine, merely escaping the wolves. As he was sliding down the vine, he heard a growl from below, only to see a pack of lions awaiting his descent. Things quickly went from bad to worse, with lions now ready to greet him at the bottom and wolves eagerly waiting for him from above. Suddenly, he heard a nibbling sound by his ear and peered up to see a mouse gnawing at the very vine that he was grasping onto with all his might.

With the wolves at the top, the lions at the bottom and a mouse gnawing at the vine, he happened to notice a plump, ripe strawberry growing out of the cliff right beside him. He reached out, plucked the strawberry from its stem and popped it into his mouth. He closed his eyes, licked his lips and savored the flavour of the most delicious strawberry he had ever tasted.

Note: This story, again, reinforces the notion that behind there may be tragedy as well as in front of us, and yet in this present moment we have the ability to taste the sweetness of life.

STUDENT REFLECTION QUESTIONS

How does this story relate to mindfulness?
    What do the wolves and the lions symbolize?
    What does the ripe, juicy strawberry symbolize?

A KOAN ON LETTING GO

One day, two monks were walking down a path leading to the Monastery. When they came to the river, they noticed that the torrential rains had washed away the bridge and that a young maiden was standing on the shore, trying to figure out how to get across. The old monk picked up the maiden, carried her across the raging river and placed her on the opposite bank. The master and his young student then continued their journey down the path. After a short while, the young monk asked the master, "Why did you pick up the young maiden, when we are forbidden to engage with women as part of our vows?" The old monk turned to the young man and said, "I left her at the river bank. Are you still carrying her?"

Note: This story helps develop a mind that lets go. It enables them to focus on things they may be ruminating on that are keeping them stuck in the past.

STUDENT REFLECTION QUESTION

What thoughts are you still carrying that it is time to let go of?

BREATHING TECHNIQUE FOR RELEASING THE PAST

- Fall out breaths, emphasize the dropping of the jaw
- Pursed lip breathing, visualizing letting go of the past with each exhalation

Movement for releasing the past
- Fall out breaths
- Standing or seated forward bends
- Downward dog
- Child's pose
- Cat/Cow building up to a vigorous pace

IS IT GOOD, OR IS IT BAD?

The following story is designed to help get away from black and white thinking, whether things are good or bad. In reality, good things can become bad and bad things can become good. We want the student to let life flow naturally from one experience to the next without clinging to the 'good' or rejecting the 'bad'. This way they can accept life and learn from the lessons embedded in all experiences.

One day, an old man was journeying through the desert and found a magnificent black Arabian stallion. It appeared to belong to no one, so he placed a rope around its neck and headed back to his village. With each step, he thanked Allah for blessing him with such an extraordinary creature and thought to himself that he must have done something right for this gift to be bestowed upon him.

At the edge of the village, he called all the people forward to show them his great find and explained that today they would slaughter his best lamb, and everyone would feast with him to celebrate this gift.

They drank and ate throughout the evening and the old man went to bed with a grateful heart, for this was one of the greatest days of his life.

The next morning, he awoke to hear his son outside, attempting to ride the stallion. As he left his hut, he witnessed his son being thrown from the horse, tumbling to the ground and breaking his leg. The old man looked in horror, for he knew that he needed his son to help him gather all of his crops at the end of the season. No one else in the village would be able to help him because they were all faced with the same task. He now looked upon the horse and cursed it as a devil and a gift from Satan, not God. He went to bed at the end of this day, with hatred in his heart, cursing the fact that the horse had ever crossed his path.

The next day, he was awakened by rebels going from hut to hut, looking for young men that they could take back with them into the hills and indoctrinate into their army When they came upon the old man's dwelling, upon entering they witnessed the young boy and his broken leg. Unfit to take with them, they left the boy behind, knowing he would only slow them down. Once again, the old man saw that the horse was a great gift from God and felt immensely blessed to have encountered this incredible creature.

QUESTION

Can you recall a moment when something was 'bad' and it became 'good' or when something was 'good' that became 'bad'?

Note: We are aiming to maintain an even perspective about all life experiences before jumping to categorize them as 'good' or 'bad'. Rather, we want to teach them that there are challenges and blessings within every situation.

We can also introduce the affirmation, "It is what it is" to encourage us to assume a balanced mind when we cannot understand or change something. This is not complacency but rather a recognition that this is the current state of reality and ruminating about it will be unproductive. "It is what it is" allows us to accept what is and move forward in the ways we can.

WRITE A HAIKU POEM

A haiku is a traditional Japanese poem comprising of three short lines that do not rhyme. The first and last lines have five syllables and the middle line has seven, known as the 5-7-5 structure.

A haiku is a wonderful assignment for a mindfulness class, since it encourages a person to look at the physical world and our human existence in a reflective manner, invoking deep emotion in the reader.

A sample haiku that reflects mindfulness teachings might read like this:
Breathing in and out,
The mind begins to slow down,
Where peace and calm live.

FIRST NATIONS MINDFULNESS PRACTICES

By Janean Marshall and Beverley Jeddore

"I AM" EXERCISE: CLAIMING YOUR IDENTITY

For the last five years, Yoga in Schools has been collaborating with the First Nations Mi'kmaw Kina'matnewey (MK) School Board spearheaded by Janean Marshall. Over this period of time, 37 teachers have been certified in the 200-hour Yoga in Schools program and 47 teachers have been trained in the Mindfulness in Schools Program. Their family of schools was the first Aboriginal School Board to offer Yoga Grade 11 as an accredited course as well as Mindfulness in North America.

We are honoured to have the input of Janean Marshall and Beverley Jeddore on these First Nations influenced mindfulness lesson plans.

The following is the way First Nations Elder Beverly Jeddore introduced herself at the beginning of the workshop she led at the Yoga in Schools Conference in Halifax. As she stated each phrase with clarity and pride, she transported us into her current reality with details of her heritage, her roles, her responsibilities and her passions.

By taking the time to fill out these open statements, we are solidifying our identity and acknowledging everyone and everything that has contributed to who we are. This is a very empowering exercise for clarifying who we are in this moment.

We have been given permission to use her personal "I AM" exercise to help inspire the writing of your own. Below you will find her version, followed by a hand out for your students to fill out on their own time. Once completed, it is suggested to have the class join in small circles and share their "I AM" exercise with their peers.

Note: with any group work that involves sharing of oneself, it is important to have agreement from participants that they will listen to their classmates' presentation with respect.

I AM …

Childhood Possessions
I am from diamonds and gems as I collected these as a passion
I am from transistor radios as I loved listening to music
I am from a tea set that my mother gave me

Food
I am from lusknikn as my mother made this on a daily basis
I am from vegetables taken from my garden
I am from beef from my farm
I am from apli'kmuj, plawej, aq nme'jk

Family
I am from Sarah Johnson and Noel R. Denny
I am the third youngest of a family of 12
I am a sister

I am an aunt to 50 nieces and nephews
I am a mother to four children two sons and two daughters
I am a grandmother to 17 grandchildren
I am a godmother to 10 godchildren
I am a widow as my husband of 38 years past away

Music
I am from the chant jukwa'luk kwe'ji'juow
I am from the Bee Gees and Lobo generation
I am a member of a choir for the past 44 years
I am a hymnal singer for Saint Ann
I am a chanter

Things in the Neighborhood
I am from a pond in my yard that I skated with my family
I am from a famous hill in QB that I was sliding on a daily basis
I am from Qamsipuk
I am from Ji ji's a store that I loved going
I am from pa'sliktuk where our cows went to eat
I am from a anklan's that I loved to play in

Family Memories
I am from the chicken coop collecting eggs
I am from the roof top as me and my sisters hung out and played
I am from the big tree in the yard that I climbed in every day
I am from a family who played the drums and played guitar
I am from travelling with our trailer to Maine, Moncton and PEI

Your Heritage
I am a member of the Denny family & Johnson family
I am from the jakej clan
I am from herbal medicines
I am from playing waltes
I am from dancing the kojua

Sayings
I am from the words: you're not the first and you won't be the last
I am from the words of love for my children & your children: kesalul tu's; kesa'lul kwi's

I AM EXERCISE: FILL IN YOUR OWN

Childhood Possessions
I am …

_____

_____

_____

Food
I am …

_____

_____

_____

Family
I am …

_____

_____

_____

Music
I am …

_____

_____

_____

Things in the Neighborhood
I am …

_____

_____

_____

Family Memories
I am …

_____

_____

_____

Your Heritage
I am …

_____

_____

_____

Sayings
I am…

_____

_____

_____

I AM …

_____

_____

_____

THE MEDICINE WHEEL

As First Nations people, we carry our medicine wheel everywhere we go, no matter what race we represent All races are included in the wheel and each have equal parts.

The medicine wheel has four directions/colors

WjipnukEast wataptek	yellow
Pkite'snukSouthmekwe'k	red
TkisnukWestmaqtewe'k	black
OqwatnukNorthwape'k	white

The medicine wheel describes your life as an individual. The first person you deal with on a daily basis is you.

Daytime

When you wake up in the morning you know that another day has been assigned to you. You prepare for the day by purifying yourself, cleansing, brushing your teeth, combing your hair and dressing. The lower part of the wheel from **East, South & West** is designed for work and leisure.

Night-time

When the day is over and the sun goes down, darkness rises and you prepare for the night in a similar fashion, by cleansing your body and preparing for sleep. Your senses, limbs, ideas, and energy must rest and be silent to feel restored for the next day's activities The upper part of the wheel, **West, North & East**, allows the body to rest.

This model provides a balance between activity and rest throughout the course of a full 24-hr cycle.

The medicine wheel depicts the life cycle of an individual:

The **East** represent life cycle of 0-7 years You have someone feeding you and taking care of you Slowly you begin to crawl, talk, and walk Hand to hand transition takes place as a parent/guardian passes the hand to a teacher It is represented by the color yellow.

The **South** represents life cycle of 7-14 years You are considered a child, which brings you to adolescence Children have greater responsibilities as they age The South is represented by the color red our nation.

The **West** represents life cycle of 14-21 years In this age category individuals are required to make plans for the future of how they would put a roof over their heads and also their career choice in life It is represented by the color black.

The **North** represents life cycle of 21-28, 28-35, 35-42 etc. We mature every 7 years and we remain here until all our hair is white. It is represented by the color white.

At the center of this wheel is where we stand, in the present moment of our lives right now.

Seven is a significant number in the Mi'kmaq tradition. We have seven Mi'kmaq districts, seven cries, seven medicines, seven worlds, seven generations etc. The most common is the seven sacred Mi'kmaq teachings which are love, humility, honesty, respect, truth, wisdom & courage. When you have these teachings, empathy is the result, which is the key component of them all. Our people naturally show great compassion in times of need especially during times of death or illness. The whole community shares your grief or suffering.

Medicine Wheel Mindful Movement Class

Ideally done outside, on a school field or playground.

Turn to face the east and do one namaskara in honor of our early childhood, visualizing the color yellow.

Turn to face the south, and do one namaskara in honor of our middle childhood, visualizing the color red.

Turn to face the west, and do one namaskara in honor of our adolescence, visualizing the color black.

Turn to face the north and do one namaskara in honor of our adulthood, visualizing the color white.

Stand in Mountain Pose and be present to your current phase of life.

Smudging Ritual

Note: it is strongly recommended to invite an Elder from your community to perform a smudging ritual, as it is a sacred practice that should be conducted by someone within the tradition.

Smudging is sacred among First Nations people We smudge our homes, ourselves, our loved ones, and our gatherings We use four sacred medicines: tobacco, sage, cedar, and sweet grass.

We begin smudging ourselves by first giving thanks to the plants who give their life force to us so that we may cleanse our bodies, minds and spirits.

We smudge each part of the body for purification, and we ask

1. Head – I ask that my thoughts, ideas, and knowledge be cleansed. I ask for blessings for my mind so that I think only kind thoughts for myself and others.
2. Eyes – I ask that my eyes be cleansed. I ask for blessings on all the things I see so that I may recognize and appreciate the beauty of Mother Earth.
3. Ears – I ask that my ears be cleansed. I ask for blessings on all the things I hear. May I listen for your whispers of guidance and use it to heal and grow.
4. Mouth – I ask that my mouth be cleansed. I ask for blessings on all the things I say so that the words I speak are truthful, kind and caring.
5. Heart – I ask that my heart be cleansed. I ask for blessings for those I love and the things I love. May I act in ways that bring more love into the world.
6. Hands – I ask that my hands be cleansed. I ask for blessings on the work I do with my hands for you, my creator. May I use my hands to touch and hold life with respect and to create beautiful things.
7. Legs/feet – I ask that my legs and feet be cleansed. I ask for blessings on the path that I travel so that my feet lead me in the direction of my true self.
8. Whole body – I ask that my whole body be cleansed of negativity so that only positive energy remains. I ask for blessings for me as a human being so that during this day you have given me, I will be able to do your work, my creator.

As humans we must know that our purpose in life is to live in peace and harmony with others. We share life with Creation and all living things These living things have a spirit and purpose in this life, just as we do. We must be taught to respect and protect all of life.

ADDITIONAL CROSS-CURRICULAR ACTIVITIES FOR INCORPORATING MINDFULNESS TEACHINGS THROUGH STORY TELLING

- Reflect on one of your life experiences that gave you a powerful lesson. Write a story about it by describing the situation, what happened and what the learning was as a result.

- Your Perfect Place: the mind is a powerful force that can either wreak havoc on our entire body-mind system by ruminating on a potentially negative outcome or contribute to our well-being by creating positive, nourishing imagery. To help guide students toward thoughts of safety that stimulate the parasympathetic nervous system (rest and digest or green zone), have them write a guided meditation whereby they visit their own special place. Encourage them to describe the journey to and from as well as their perfect place in great detail, with the two-fold goal of calming their own minds and also sharing their special place with others. Some examples might be a secluded beach, a forest walk, a hike up to a mountain peak, a cozy private room with a beautiful view etc.

- Your Future Self: write a story about your ideal future self, describing who you are, how you spend your time, what gifts you contribute to the world and what brings you joy.

- Letter to your future self: reflect on three questions you currently have about your life and write a letter to your future self, asking the questions that you seek answers to. Leave space below each question so that you can record the answers as they arise. You can also write a letter from your future self to your current self, imagining what support s/he would give you, or simply offer three supportive statements from your future self to your current self that reassure any fears, anxieties or uncertainties you have about your future.

- Write a children's story that is themed on a mindfulness principle, add photos or illustrations and present it to your classmates and/or read it to a younger book buddy.

- Select a music video that tells a story about challenge, suffering, growth and understanding. Write a report on it, answering why you chose this video, what life lesson it tells, and how it inspires you in your own life.

- Drama activity #1: Freeze Frame. In small groups of five or six, create a five-part vignette of one of the aspects of mindfulness, such as turning away from negative thoughts to more helpful thought patterns, or shifting from doing to being, from consumerism to contentment etc.

- Drama activity #2: Human Machine. In small groups, create a machine or function related to mindfulness, being sure to include each person in your group. Some suggestions might be the workings of the triune brain, including the pre-frontal cortex, the hippocampus and the amygdala, or people communicating mindfully, or the lungs breathing etc.

- Write up a daily mindfulness schedule, which includes how you wake up, what you do to start your day (what you do first thing in the morning sets the pace and tone for the rest of your day), mindful breaks, meal-time routine, social engagements, and end of day rituals for sleep preparation. This is an excellent time-management exercise and helps students become more aware of how they spend each moment.

MINDFULNESS AND SCHOOL-WIDE INITIATIVES

Mindfulness can be practiced as an individual, as a family, as a classroom and as a school. The following are but a few suggestions for sharing the gifts of mindfulness with your entire student body:

- Meditation in the morning over the loud speaker with the whole school to start the day in the green zone.
- Replace the schools loud buzzing bell with mindfulness chimes or gentle music as a reminder to not only change classes but to enjoy three deep cleansing breaths.
- Have a school-wide Mindfulness Manifesto, where kids research an aspect of mindfulness and exhibit their work in booths for the whole school to peruse. Booths could include painting rocks, coloring mandalas, aromatherapy for calming the body/mind, knitting as a mindfulness practice, nature/focusing walk, drumming, attention exercises like looking at a plate of 10 items for 30 seconds and then write down everything you remember afterward.
- Create a Mindfulness Day to complement winter carnival.
- Older students could teach Mindfulness to little ones, creating crafts and board games etc.

CONCLUSION
BECOMING PART OF THE SOLUTION THROUGH MINDFUL ACTION

From a global standpoint, planet earth is teetering on a tipping point, where humans must change the way we are living or face self-destruction with the ever-pressing reality of climate change. It is undeniable now that the earth is heating up, our forests are disappearing, and our oceans are rising. But the same human species that got us into this mess can also get us out, and a mindful lifestyle can take us from being part of the problem to becoming the solution.

As mindfulness teacher David A. Treleavan says "We need to differentiate between the mind state of mindfulness and taking mindful action in the world." While an individual mindfulness practice encourages a neutral, unbiased observation of life as it is, the moment we engage in our lives, we are taking action in some way. Even if we choose not to act, it's still an action, albeit a passive one. If action is unavoidable then, our challenge is to take thoughtful action.

Taking mindfulness into the world means that we realize that what we do (actively) or don't do (passively) all makes a difference. For example, passively observing elections without voting can have, as we've seen, catastrophic results. Therefore, realizing that what we do and even what we don't do matters, we must consider our stance and the power we hold and then take action in a way that aligns with our core values. This is mindful action.

Just as we have the capacity to affect positive change within our minds, we can do the same on a global scale by becoming more conscious of our lifestyle choices. For example, knowing that industrial farming is a massive contributor to greenhouse gases, simply becoming more mindful of what we eat and where we buy our food can make a big difference.

Knowing that our planet is now inundated with chemicals that the human body has never been exposed to before and causing life-threatening allergies, illnesses and diseases, we can make mindful choices about the products we endorse. Mindfully scanning labels on packaged food, cosmetics and cleaning agents for toxic chemicals and choosing to consume non-harmful products can decrease the vast amounts of chemicals being dumped into our waterways Mindful action can affect great change with regards to the lethal synthetic chemicals used to make everything from takeout containers, to store receipts, to children's toys, to furniture and even clothing.

In the western world, it is easy to become myopically focused on our first world issues and champagne problems, spending hours primping in front of the mirror, or fighting it out in fortnite, or climbing the social ladder on social media As was discussed in class six of the mindfulness program, mindfulness has the potential to expand our awareness to include the lives of others, like the suffering of those around the planet who are surviving in war-torn situations or who wake up to the realities of severe food and water shortage each day.

If we all lived with the same perspective of our First Nations people, who believe that every action we make has the potential to affect the next seven generations, we might all become more mindful of how we spend our precious moments.

As David Suzuki once said "In a world of more than seven billion people, each of us is a drop in the bucket. But with enough drops, we can fill any bucket." We all have the opportunity and the responsibility to live our lives more mindfully, and as we do, we all win.

Let's be the change,

Jenny and **Blair**

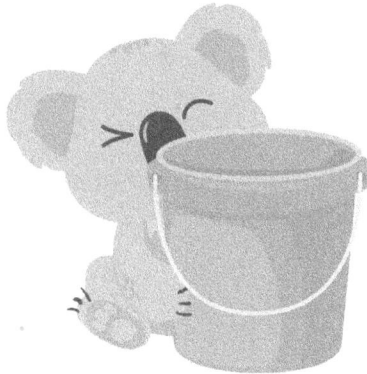

Bye for now friends!
Remember to Relax, Breath and Choose.

References and Resources

The following list of materials are referenced in this manual or may be used for further study.

Elizabeth Blackburn, *The Telomere Effect—the new science of living younger* (Grand Central Publishing, 2017)

Tara Brach, *Radical Acceptance—embracing your life with the heart of a Buddha* (Random House Canada, 2004)

Pema Chodron, *When things fall apart – heart advise for difficult times* (Shambhala, 2016)

Deepak Chopra, *Super Brain—unleashing the explosive power of your mind to maximize health,* (Harmony, 2012)

Mark Coleman, *Make Peace with your Mind—How mindfulness and compassion can free you from your inner critic,* (New World Library, 2016)

Nancy Colier, The Power of OFF—the mindful way to stay sane in a virtual world (Sounds True, 2016)

Ram Dass, *Be Here Now* (Harmony, 1971)

Viktor Frankl, Man's Search for Meaning, (Beacon Press, 2006)

William Glasser, *Choice Theory: A new Psychology of Personal Freedom,* (HarperCollins Publishers, 1999)

Thich Nhat Hanh, *The Miracle of Mindfulness* (Beacon Press, 1996) and *A Handful of Quiet,* (Plum Blossom, 2008)

Steven Handel, Mindfulness and Neuroplasticity, http://www.theemotionmachine.com/mindfulness-and-neuroplasticity (Posted on May 17, 2011)

Rick Hanson, *Buddha's Brain—the practical neuroscience of happiness, love and wisdom,* (New Harbinger Publications, 2009) and *Resilient—how to grow an unshakable core of calm, strength and happiness* (Harmony, 2018)

Donald Hebb, *The organization of behavior* (John Wiley & Sons Inc, 1754)

Pierce J. Howard, *The Owner's Manual for the Brain* (William Morrow, 2014)

Tom Ireland, *Scientific American* "What does mindfulness meditation do to your brain". https://blogs.scientificamerican.com/guest-blog/what-does-mindfulness-meditation-do-to-your-brain (June 12, 2014)

Frances E. Jensen, *The Teenage Brain* (Collins, 2015)

Kachan D, Olano H, Tannenbaum SL, Annane DW, Mehta A, Arheart KL, et al. Prevalence of Mindfulness Practices in the US Workforce: National Health Interview Survey. Prev Chronic Dis 2017;14:160034. DOI: http://dx.doi.org/10.5888/pcd14.160034

Jack Kornfield, *A Path with Heart—a guide through the perils and promises of spiritual life,* (Bantam, 2009)

Leah Kuypers, *Zones of Regulation—a curriculum designed to foster self-regulation and emotional control* (Think Social Publishing, 2011)

Kelly J. Mahler, I*nteroception—the eighth sensory system,* (Aapc Publishing, 2015)

Sue McGreevey, *Mindfulness Meditation training Changes Brain Structure in Just 8 Weeks* http://www.massgeneral.org/about/pressrelease.aspx?id=1329 (January 21, 2011)

Michael Meade, *Men and The Water of Life: Initiation and the Tempering of Men,* (San Francisco: Harper, 1994)

Sarah Montana, Ted Talk, *The Real Risk of Forgiveness–And Why It's Worth It,* https://www.youtube.com/watch?v=mEK2pIiZ2I0

Dr. Kristin Neff, Self-Com*passion—the proven power of being kind to yourself* (William Morrow Paperback, 2015)

M. Scott M.D. Peck, *The Road Less Travelled—a new psychology of love, tranditional values and spiritual growth* (Touchstone, 2003)

Daniel Rechtschaffen, *The Way of Mindful Education – Cultivating Well Being in Teachers and Students* (WW Norton, 2014)

Sharon Salzberg, *Loving Kindness and Real Happiness* (Shambhala, 2002)

Daniel J. Siegal MD, *Brain Storm—the power and purpose of the teenage brain,*

(TarcherPerigee, 2014) and The Developing Mind (The Guilford Press, 2015)

Daniel J Seigel MD and Tina Payne Bryson PhD, *The Whole Brain Child* (Bantam, 2012)

Irene Smit and Astrid van der Hulst, *A Book That Takes It's Time—an unhurried adventure in Creative Mindfulness,* (Workman Publishing Company, 2017)

Eline Snel, *Sitting Still Like a Frog—mindfulness exercises for kids* (Shambhala, 2013)

Eckhart Tolle, *The Power of NOW—a guide to spiritual enlightenment* (New World Library, 2004)

David A. Treleaven, *Trauma-Sensitive Mindfulness—Practices for safe and transformative healing* (WW Norton, 2018)

Jon Kabat Zinn, *Full Catastrophe Living—using the wisdom of your body and mind to face stress, pain and illness* (Random House Publishing Group, 2013) and *Coming to our Senses—healing ourselves and the world through mindfulness* (Hachette Books, 2006

www.ingramcontent.com/pod-product-compliance
Lightning Source LLC
Chambersburg PA
CBHW080621030426

42336CB00018B/3036